普通の精神科医？
―うつ病の闇への航海―

著　　　　明　　海
写真・解説　マーク・ソープ
翻　訳　　　リー・ダンシー

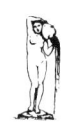

星 和 書 店

Seiwa Shoten Publishers

2-5 Kamitakaido 1-Chome
Suginamiku Tokyo 168-0074, Japan

少し長いまえがき

これは、精神科医がうつ病になった話である。この本の内容から、うつ病の経過がどのようなものかおわかりいただけると思う。うつ病の迷路をそのままたどると時間は前後し、道のりも混迷して、あまりに複雑だ。そこで、経過をわかりやすくするため、最初に少し長いまえがきにお付き合いいただければ幸いである。

うつ病になった精神科医とは私のことである。二十年近い臨床経験があり、教育や研究にも従事してきた。医師は自分の専門分野の病気になるというジンクスがあるが、それはまじめな研究者のことであって、他人事だと思っていた。それでも、もし精神疾患になることがあったら……と考え、うつ病にはなりたくないと思ったものである。うつ病の人は見るからに苦しそうだったから。

ところが、こともあろうに、一番なりたくなかったうつ病におびやかされることになってしまった。慢性的な疲労が続いていたうえ、立て続けに強いストレスにさらされて、うつ病

の罠にはまってしまった。実に巧妙な罠であった。

最初は自分が罠にはまり込んだことに気づかなかった。何かが違うと感じただけだった。疲れやすく、眠れず、集中力もなくなってきたが、まさかうつ病になりかけているのだとは思わなかった。忙しいし、とにかく仕事、仕事……と思っているうちに、気持ちが沈んで不安が強くなった。決断しなければならないことが決められず、くよくよ悩む。それでも、まあそのうち何とかなるだろうと思って放っておいたら、ますますひどくなって仕事や日常生活に影響が出始めた。

これはまずい、うつ状態かもしれないと考えて抗うつ薬をのみ始めた。薬さえのめばよくなるはずだと思った。

ほんの数日間しか処方されない風邪薬さえのみ忘れるのが常で、ドクターの指示は全然守らない勝手な患者であった私にしては、めずらしく殊勝な心がけであった。それだけ切羽詰まっていたということでもある。ひとまず、治療は薬に任せて仕事を続けた。とにかく忙しいし、具合が悪くなっている暇なんかないというわけだ。ところが、そこに友人が突然亡く

なるという強いストレスが加わるに及んで、症状は真っ逆さまに転落するように悪化し、とうとう仕事が続けられなくなった。

退職してアルバイトだけをすることにしたが、それでも症状はなかなか改善しない。もしかすると抗うつ薬の副作用をうつ病の症状を勘違いしているのかもしれないと解釈して、抗うつ薬を中断してしまった。もはや物事を理論的、客観的に考えることができなくなっていた。服薬を中断したら症状はさらに悪化してしまい、そこでようやく服薬していた薬の効果に気づく始末である。そして、やはり薬物療法は必要であるという結論に至るのだが、副作用のでる薬をもう一度のみ始めるのはどうにも気が進まなかった。そこで違う抗うつ薬に変更してみた。治療薬を変えて、多少症状がよくなってきたが、よい状態は長続きしなかった。少し楽になったかと思うとまた悪くなり、暴風雨の海か、激しいスコールの来る夜のジャングル（行ったことはないが）顔負けの状態である。

不安定な状態に疲労困憊して投げやりになってきたとき、友人たちが助けてくれた。彼らの助けがあったからこそ、時間が経つのを待つことができた。友人たちの優しいサポート、休養、薬物治療の三つがそろってようやく、うつ病の暗い迷路から脱出することができたの

だと思う。そして、一年以上の月日を経て、新しい仕事に就き、新しい仲間ができ、何とかまた生活していくことができるようになった。

未だに、自分が生存しているのかどうかさえ不確かに感じられ、何のために生きているのかと余計な考えにとらわれることもある。しかし、うつ病を経験しなければ、生涯めぐりあうことのなかったであろう、素晴らしい人々と出会い、生涯理解することのできなかったであろう、貴重な智慧を身につけることができた。

編集者の曽根氏には、本文中に会話を増やしたほうが読みやすいとアドバイス頂いた。何日も何日も考えたが、会話を思い出すことができない。というか、具合が悪かった当時、実際に会話をすることさえ困難であったし、内容も覚えていられなかった。自分の内面で荒れ狂っている嵐に圧倒され、その嵐に打ち負かされないよう、ひたすら身を縮めているのが精一杯であった。

この本の原稿を書き始めたのは、退職はしたものの、まだ症状が不安定であった頃、抗うつ薬を変更する前からである。そのため、特に前半部分は文章自体が理解しにくく、悲観的

で単調なところが多い。後半部分に移るにしたがって、希望がみえ始め、文章にも多少のめりはりが出てくることに気づいていただけることと思う。文体そのものにもうつ病の症状である思考障害が反映されているため、あえて読者に読みやすいように変更することは避けることにした。ご理解いただければ幸いである。

それでは、うつ病の迷路へご案内しよう。ガイド付きなので、出口がみつからないのではないかという心配は杞憂である。

明　海

この本を手にとられた方へ

> この本は、うつ病についての医学的な解説書ではありません。一つの症例の経過を見ていくことにより、うつ病の症状について知っていただくこと、また、うつ病は回復する障害であることを知っていただくことを目的としたものです。

あなたがもしうつ病の診断を受けておられるのであれば

- 無理をしないでお読みください。数行読んで疲れてしまうようなら、あるいは読もうとしても気力がなくなってしまうようなら、読むのは一度やめましょう。数週間経ってからまた、ページを開いてみてください。

- あなたが今、生きていることさえつらいと感じていても、決して死を選んではなりません。現在の状態は必ず変化していきます。あなたは、つらい状態を治療者や周

りの人に伝えていますか。まだ伝えていないのなら、必ずあなたの状態を彼らに知らせて、助けを求めてください。苦しいときに助けを求めることをためらわないでください。彼らは必ず、あなたの力になってくれるでしょう。

あなたがもしうつ病の患者さんのご家族や友人であるなら

- うつ病の症状について理解してください。この本に出てくる症状は、比較的典型的な症状ですが、人によって、もっと軽い場合も、重い場合もあります。症状がある程度以上重くなると、患者さんは症状を訴えたり、自覚したりすることも難しくなります。患者さんの言動を見ていて心配であれば、苦しいことがあるかどうか、ご本人に確認してください。また、患者さんがうつ病の症状や、治療薬の効果・副作用について治療者に十分説明できないような状態であれば、診察に付き添って、患者さんにかわり、治療者に状況を伝えてください。

- 患者さんが自分は治らないのではないかと心配しているときは、うつ病は必ず回復する障害であることをくり返し伝えてください。そして、焦らずに休養と治療を続

けるよう話してください。

- 元気なときにできていたことができなくなっているとき、患者さんを励ましたり、叱咤激励したりしないでください。うつ病は、気合いを入れれば治るというものではありません。また、患者さんが怠けているから物事ができないわけでもありません。それはうつ病の症状の一つであり、治療が必要な状態なのです。

- うつ病は、通常数カ月の治療で回復することが多いのですが、場合によっては経過が長引くことがあります。側で見ているのはつらいでしょうが、どうか焦らないでください。

- うつ病にはイライラ感がよく見られます。場合によっては患者さんがあなたに当たり散らしたり、あなたを傷つけたりするようなことを言うかもしれません。しかしそれは、元気なときのその人の言動とは違うのではありませんか。患者さんの症状に巻き込まれず、冷静になってください。

● あなたがうつ病の患者さんやそのご家族、友人以外の方であれば

あなたがこの本を手にとられた理由は何でしょうか。もしかして、うつ病かもしれない、と思われるのでしたら、専門家にご相談ください。精神科や心療内科を受診することは決して恥ずかしいことではありません。あなたは腹痛がひどいとき、病院に行くのをためらったりするでしょうか。

● ちょっと興味があるからページをめくってみたという方。お手にとっていただいてありがとうございます。うつ病は頻度の高い疾患です。実際に経験するかどうかは別として、誰にでもうつ病になるリスクはあるのです。これを機会にうつ病について知っていただき、ひいては精神疾患への偏見を（もしおもちであれば）なくしていただきたいと思います。

目次

少し長いまえがき iii

この本を手にとられた方へ viii

1 三万五千フィート上空での回想 1

2 きっかけ 3

3 抗うつ薬 6

4 生活上の支障 11

5 精神科受診 16

6 身体の病気？ 18

7 うつ病の認識 20

8 気持ちの沈み 22

9 悲観 25

10 自殺 26

11 判断の誤り	31
12 断酒	34
13 ジェットコースター	37
14 たどりつけない迷路の出口	41
15 鯨をめぐる旅	48
16 信頼	55
17 ある日の朝	56
18 笑う	63
19 存在の支え	68
20 エピローグ	71

● 反射光──マーク・ソープ 75

● 迷い込んだ不死鳥──倉田 洋二 83

あとがき 87

翻訳者からのメッセージ 91

1 三万五千フィート上空での回想

「精神科医になるには……」

医学部キャンパスの中の、窓がなく、広いとも言えないその部屋の中で、当時学生だった私は話していた。

「適性に欠けるような気がします、自分は。学問としてはとても面白いんですが、これまで何不自由なく過ごしてきてしまって、大変な経験をしたこともないので……、患者さんのことがよく理解できないんじゃないかと……」

私の向かい側に座っていたカウンセラーは、精神科医になるために患者の苦痛を経験する必要はないし、何不自由なく過ごしてきたのなら今この部屋にいないのではないか、と指摘した。まあ、当然の指摘だ。

もう外は暗くなっている頃だろう。そろそろ退出する時間であった。

結局、私は精神科医になった。そして二十年後、講演の開催地へ向かう飛行機の中で、長い間記憶の底に埋もれていた、あの狭く殺風景な部屋の中での会話が静かに蘇った。

こんなに長く精神科医をやっているのに、その間に多くの症例を経験してきたのに、うつ病の症状さえ何も理解していなかった。この数カ月、自分が苦しんでいる状況は、何も理解しないでここまで来てしまった代償なのだ、おそらくは。自分の愚かさがどうしようもなく悔やまれる。それに、このひどい頭の重さと疲労感は、いったいどうすればよいのだろうか。これから三時間の講演など、とてもできそうにない。いっそ、このまま飛行機が墜落してくれたらどんなに楽だろうか。

しかし重い頭の芯ではまた別のことを考えていた。うつ病の症状や経過を熟知している自分でさえ実際にこれだけ苦痛なのだから、医学的な知識のない患者さんはどんなに不安だろうか。よくこの状態を乗り切れるものだと、苦しい状況を耐え忍ぶ姿に頭が下がった。うつ病にみられる気持ちの落ち込みは、普通の人の気持ちの落ち込みの程度の重いものだと説明されることがあるが、それは全然違う。症状を経験したことのない家族や友人、職場の同僚に理解してもらうのは、ほとんど無理だろう。苦しい症状の中で、もう自分は治らないのではないかと思ってしまう。

誰かが患者さんにかわって周囲の人々に症状を説明することができたら、助けになるかも

しれない。それよりもまず、訳がわからないうちにのみ込まれてしまったにちがいない症状の内容を患者さん自身に少しでも知らせることができたら、多少は安心できるのではないだろうか。それをするのに、うつ病になった精神科医以上の適役はいないと考えていた。

この本は、精神科医である私が実際に体験したうつ病についての記録であり、カタルシスを目的とした私小説ではない。背景や詳細は多少修飾してあるが、うつ病についての記載は実体験に基づいている。

2 きっかけ

うつ病を発症するきっかけは、「これさえなければ、精神科に来ることもなかったのに」という、はっきりした原因があることもあるが、原因が明らかでない場合もある。私の場合は、親しい友人の死がうつ病の最後の引き金を引いた。その別れは二年続けて起こり、いずれもあまりに突然で、何の心の準備もできなかった。二度目の友人の死は私を決定的に打ち

のめしたが、最初の友人の死の一年ほど前から、すでにうつ病の準備状態とでもいうべき状況にあった。その当時、私はある医療機関で教育と研究に携わり、付属の医療機関で臨床指導医として働いていた。

四月に最初の友人を失った年は仕事の内容も多岐にわたり、ひどく疲れるようになった。仕事を終えて帰宅すると、もうひと言もしゃべる元気さえなかった。食事も作れず、家の近くのデリでサンドイッチを買ってきた。食べ物を選ぶことも面倒なのでいつも同じ、ホールウィートにハムとチーズ、ホワイトブレッドにエッグサラダという組み合わせになった。ビールを飲んで、買ってきたものを少し食べると、身体を起こしていることができず、そのままカーペットの上で横になった。着替えて顔を洗ってベッドに入るという作業の前に、まず休まなければならないのであった。

その当時はまだ睡眠をとることができたが、朝起きると途方もなく疲れていた。眠ったのだから疲れは多少とれているはずなのに、前の晩ベッドに入ったときよりもっと疲れている感じである。とても仕事に行けそうにないと思う。そのため、職場に電話をして仕事を休むという誘惑と延々と戦わなければならなかった。「体調が悪いので」「熱があるので」「めま

いがするので」「ひどい風邪を引いたので」という言い訳を頭の中で反芻するが、どれも説得力がなかった。そんなことぐらいで私が休むはずがないことは誰もが知っている。足の骨折以外は絶対に仕事を休んではならないという教育を受けてきた私は、二十年間のうち当日の病欠は五日ぐらいだったと思う。病院で働くには、ある一時期猛烈に働いて、そのあとに倒れるなどということは許されない。最も大切なのは、心身ともに一定の良好なレベルでコンスタントに働き続けるということである。しかもできるだけ長時間。

そのときの私には、一日休んだぐらいでは疲労がとれないことがおぼろげながらわかっていた。一日でも休んでしまえば、おそらく何日も休むことになるだろう。休んだときに同僚にかかる迷惑や、その日にこなさなければならない会議やアポイントメント、翌日に仕事量がさらに増えることを考えると、電話をかけて休むこと自体も苦痛に思えてきた。

何としても出勤しなければならないと決心するとベッドを出るのだが、そのままクローゼットの前に座り込んで動けなくなってしまう。着るものが決められないのだ。顔を洗うにも疲れきっていて、洗面台に身体をもたせかけなければならなかった。

もともと朝型で、早朝に仕事を始める習慣がある私の出勤時間は徐々に遅くなった。遅刻をするようなことはなかったが、何よりも朝がつらかった。出勤するか休むか、朝の自分との戦いは毎日、何週間にもわたって続いた。一応専門家である私には、朝にひどく具合が悪いということは何を意味するのかを知っていた。うつ状態である。

3　抗うつ薬

とにかく、何とかしなければならなかった。うつ状態の治療は、原因のあるなしにかかわらず、基本的には同じである。抗うつ薬を用いた薬物療法と休養が車の両輪のように、ともに重要であると、どの教科書や解説書にも書いてある。しかし、それと同じくらい大切なのは周囲からのサポートであることに、私はまだ気づいていなかった。そのことがわかったのは、仕事ができなくなって、さらに何カ月もたってからのことであった。とりあえず、抗うつ薬に話を戻そう。

抗うつ薬にはいろいろな種類がある。薬物療法を専門としてきたため、私は何種類かの抗うつ薬を服用した経験があった。効果を確認するためではなく、副作用を経験するためである。自分で実際に薬を服用したほうが患者さんにわかりやすく説明できるし、彼らに何を質問すればよいのかもわかってくる。

抗うつ薬は効果が現れるまでに時間がかかる。早くて数日から一週間、場合によっては一カ月近くかかることもある。一方、副作用は人によって、あるいは服用量によって出現したりしなかったりするが、出現するときには服用後数日以内に出てくることが多い。だから、抗うつ薬を服用するときには、効果が出てくるのを待つ間、副作用を我慢しなければならないことになる。気持ちが落ち込んでいて、気力がなく、話をすることもおっくうな患者さんは、副作用が出ていても、それすら治療者に言わず、自分の判断で服薬を中止してしまうことがある。そのため、抗うつ薬を処方し始めた初期は特に、治療者のほうが副作用や効果について細かく聞かなければならない。あるいは、付き添ってきた家族や友人が副作用や効果が出ていると感じるときは、患者さんに代わって治療者にそれを伝えることが望ましい。

薬物治療が必要であると判断した私は、数ある抗うつ薬から、あまり副作用が強くなく効果の発現が早いとされているものを選んで服用し始めた。服用して数日間は軽い吐き気があったが、我慢できないというほどのものでもなかった。二週間ほどすると、少し気力が戻り、効果が出始めたことが実感できて、ひと安心した。これで秋の学会シーズンまで働くことができそうだし、それが過ぎれば多少は仕事量が減るから大丈夫だろうと思った。

その年は例年と比較にならないほど忙しく、通常の何倍もの仕事量をこなした。自分の状態を完全に甘くみていたのだ。休養をとらないので、多少気力が出てきたのもつかの間、また調子が悪くなった。抗うつ薬の量を増やして何とか乗り切ろうとしたが、めまいや吐き気などの副作用のため、そうすることができなかった。

抗うつ薬の服用を続けていても、症状は消えるところまではいかず、そのうちに副作用が強く感じられるようになった。抗うつ薬を服用し始めるときは、うつ病の症状がある程度重いので、多少副作用があっても楽になりたい一心でそれに耐えることは比較的容易である。

その後、症状が軽くなってくると、副作用が強く感じられるようになることがある。

服薬開始後六カ月ほどたったとき、私はいい加減服薬にうんざりしてきた。そして、症状

が改善したから副作用が気になり始めたのだと解釈し、抗うつ薬を中断してしまった。残念ながら私の判断は大きな勘違いであった。一～二週間すると、気力が全くなくなって、ひどく疲れるようになった。症状を完全に消失させないまでも、その抗うつ薬は明らかに効果を発揮していたのだ。

抗うつ薬の服用期間は、症状が改善してから四～六カ月間必要であるといわれている。早すぎる服薬の中断は、症状の再燃（一度消失した症状が再び現れること）につながる。症状が充分改善しないうちに服薬をやめてしまったので、私の症状はまた悪くなった。しかし、服薬をやめたときは、症状が一進一退の状態が長く続いており、本当にもう、薬をのむこと自体がいやだったのだ。副作用だけ残っているとしたら、服用を中止したほうが症状が良くなるかもしれないとも思った。

症状がまた悪化し、気持ちの沈み、不安感、イライラ感、意欲のなさなどが強くなったため、抗うつ薬をのみ始める必要があった。以前に服用していた薬は効果がはっきりしないうえに副作用もあって増量することもできなかった。そこで薬を変更することにした。

新しい薬に変えて数日すると、信じられないぐらいイライラ感と不安感が消え、パートタ

イムの仕事のない日は家で一日過ごすことができるようになった。意欲や集中力は完全には元に戻っていないし、時によっては症状が一時的に悪くなったように感じることもあるが、二番目に試した抗うつ薬は最初に服用した薬よりも、うつ病の症状の改善に役立っているようであった。

　私の服用した抗うつ薬の名前は、次のような理由から、あえて書かないでおこうと思う。抗うつ薬にはいくつかの系統があり、多くの薬剤が使用可能だが、どの薬剤が効果を現すかは人によって異なる。一つの抗うつ薬が有効である確率は五〇～七〇％程度である。百人の患者さんが服用したとして、五十～七十人はその薬で症状が改善するということである。この数字を見て、有効性が低いと感じる人もいるであろうが、どの抗うつ薬もこの程度の有効性であり、プラセボ（有効成分を含まない錠剤）を服用した場合に比べれば明らかに効果は優れている。どの抗うつ薬も（抗うつ薬に限らずすべての治療薬は）臨床試験によって科学的に効果や副作用が確認されている。有効率が五〇～七〇％だとしても、もしある患者さんがその薬を服用してうつ病が治れば、その人にとって薬の効果は一〇〇％であると感じられるだろう。

問題は、誰が五十～七十人の中に入るのか、前もって知ることができないことにある。トライ・アンド・エラーといって、その人の症状、年齢、病歴、身体合併症から有効性の高そうな薬を試していくしかない。したがって、私が服用して効果があったからといって、すべての人に同じ薬が有効であるとは限らない。また、副作用にしても、私の場合は増量できなかったが、私が服用した用量の何倍かの量を副作用なしに服用することができて、それで症状が良くなる人もいる。

抗うつ薬を服用するうえで大切なことは、効果が出るまでには時間がかかること、不規則な服用は意味がないので決められた量を決められたとおり服用すること、自己判断で服薬を中断しないこと、そして効果と副作用について治療者とよく話し合うこと、である。

4　生活上の支障

最初に友人が亡くなった年、秋の学会シーズンが終わって仕事が一段落した頃から、私の

気分はますます沈むようになった。このときはすでに最初の抗うつ薬を服用していたにもかかわらず。自分の診療に対するポリシーと病院の新しい運営方針が嚙み合わないこともあり、仕事に対するモチベーションがなくなっていった。巨大な病院組織の中で、私一人が異を唱えても始まらないことであった。組織の方針に同調できなければ去るしか道はない。さらに、長年私を悩ませ続けてきた私生活上の問題もますます複雑になった。どの問題をとっても自分の努力では解決することができない現実が、私を疲弊させた。

　まだ研修医の頃、例のごとく、医師という仕事が自分に合わないのではないかと悩み始めた私は、スランプに陥って壁を乗り越えられないと先輩に相談したことがあった。優秀な麻酔科医であったその先輩は、
「君は壁を乗り越えるようなタイプじゃない、壁を突き崩して進む人だ。スランプなんて冗談だろう」
と一笑した。もともとプライベートな問題を他人に相談する習慣がないので、話の内容が抽象的すぎたのかもしれない。それはともかく、壁を突き崩すと言われたパワフルな私が、自分の力が及ばない今回ばかりはどうすることもできなかった。

そして、二人目の友人が翌年の春に亡くなって、さらに打撃は決定的なものとなった。あまりにも突然の死であった。二人のとても大切な友人を二年続けてなくした衝撃は強すぎた。このまま仕事を続けていくことに限界が来たことが私にはわかった。

そして、異常な感覚がやってくるようになった。自分が別の世界に来てしまったのではないかと思えてくる。いくつもの世界が並行して存在しているような感じで、本当の世界は別のところにあり、そこではまだ友人が生きているはずなのだが、自分だけが何かとんでもない間違いで、今いる世界に迷い込んでしまった、という感覚である。

この感じは「胡蝶の夢」を連想させた。胡蝶の夢というのは、紀元前三～四世紀、中国の戦国時代に宋の国の思想家であった荘子のみた夢の話である。荘子は夢の中で蝶になり、ひらひらと舞っていた。そして目覚めたあとに考えた。自分は胡蝶の夢が現実なのか。もしかしたら胡蝶が人間になった夢をみていて、今の自分は胡蝶のみている夢の中の存在ではないだろうか。どちらが真実なのだろうかと考える、という話である。とにかくすべてが非現実的で、自分の心が身体から出ていって、数十センチメートル離れたところに浮いているような感じがした。離人感という症状である。

また、友人が亡くなったのは水曜日であったが、毎週水曜日になると、朝からひどい不安感に苛まれるようになった。友人の死を知らせる電話がまたかかってくるのではないか、この破滅的な状況がまた最初からくり返されるのではないかと思えてくる。そうすると、居てもたってもいられなくなり、じっとしていられない。さらに、記憶が曖昧になってきた。もともと私は、いつ誰に会ってどのような話をしたのかをきちんと覚えているほうなのだが、それがよく思い出せない。一日前、二日前のことさえ曖昧で、こんなにひどい物忘れが始まるとは、まさか認知症の始まりではないか、と本気で心配になった。人との約束も覚えていられないので、手帳に細かく書き込まなければならなかった。

また、人と会ったり話をしたりすることがとても苦痛になった。家にいるときは電話が怖くなった。誰からかかってきているかわからない怖さ、何か不吉なことを知らせる内容ではないかという怖さ、電話の相手の顔が見えない怖さ、話の内容が理解できないのではないかという怖さ、話の最中に自分が泣き出すのではないかという怖さ。私は電話に出ることができなくなった。留守番電話が応答し、自分はぼうっとそれを聞いているだけであった。テレビを見ることもできなくなった。特にニュースでは毎日のように、テロ、凶悪事件、自然災

害が報道される。その映像を見るだけで、不安が高まり動悸が強くなった。

電子メールのやりとりも苦痛になり、仕事上、とても困った事態を引き起こした。受信したメールが長文だったり、内容が複雑だったりすると、読む気にもならないし、実際に最後まで読めない。内容も理解できない。返信もおっくうでできない。自分でも信じられなかったが、五行以上のメールは読むのも返信するのも無理になった。しかたがないので、こちらから電話をして用事をすませましたが、電話をかけるのにまた労力が必要なのだった。

あの状態で外来勤務がこなせたのには、我ながら驚きである。安定している再診の患者さんは問題ないのだが、症状が不安定な患者さんや初診の診察にますます時間がかかり、自分の判断に誤りがないかと四六時中不安に苛まれた。

とうとう私の状態は辞職せざるを得ないところまで来てしまった。休職したらどうかと言ってくれる人もいたが、たとえ短期間であっても、私のポストで休職することは自分自身が許せなかった。

5　精神科受診

　私は年度末に退職することにした。有給休暇を使って何日か休むことにしたが、それでも最後まで働けるかどうか自信がなかった。普通ならこの時点で精神科を受診して、専門的な治療を開始すべきときである。しかし、何しろ自分自身が精神科医である。いったい誰に治療を頼めばよいのか。結局、先輩の酒井先生に、休職しなければならないときに備えて診断書を書いてもらい、自分に適当と思われる抗うつ薬を処方してもらった。診断書はとうとう使わずじまいだった。

　私が継続的に専門家に治療を依頼しなかったのには理由があった。精神科医であれば、誰でもうつ病の治療に際して、薬物療法とともに精神療法的なアプローチを用いる。うつ病のきっかけに心理的な要因があるのか、ないのか、を確かめるとともに、もし心理的ストレスがあれば、それに対処する方策を考えるのが普通である。

　私の場合、うつ病を発症するきっかけに仕事上や日常生活上のストレスが関係していた。一方で、私には職務上、いろいろな秘守義務、すなわち他人に話してはならない情報があっ

た。しかし、もし治療を受けて、親切丁寧に質問されたら、本当は話すべきでないこと、あるいは話してはならないことまで自分がしゃべるのではないか、という不安をぬぐい去れなかった。私の治療者になる精神科医にも秘守義務はあるのだから、理論的には何を話しても心配ないはずであるが、私は疑心暗鬼になっており、同業者の誰も信用できなくなっていた。診療録に詳しく自分のことを記載されるのもいやだった。クリニックならまだしも、病院を受診すれば、担当医以外にもそこに勤務している精神科医に出会うかもしれない。保険証を見れば、私の勤務先は医療スタッフにもわかってしまう。

沈み込んでいる私の様子を見た英国人医師のD先生は、知り合いの精神科医を紹介するから米国で治療を受けたらどうか、とアドバイスしてくださった。しかし、それにしても何カ月もかかるはずであり、とても渡米の準備はできそうになかった。

さらに、この期に及んでも、自分がうつ病になったとは認めたくなかった。そんな自分は許せない気がした。自分がうつ病であることをはっきり認識せざるを得なくなったのは、退職してしばらくたってからであった。

私は、第三者である専門家に治療を受けることはなかったが、このようなケースは特殊で

6 身体の病気？

病院を退職するにあたって、何人かの後輩やナースが一緒に食事をしたいと言ってくれた。その日は五人でイタリアンレストランに行くことになっていた。私は自分の車を運転して、二人のナースと一緒に予約時間どおりにレストランに着いた。後輩の一人は、他の病院から遅れてやってきた。彼が到着して席に着いたとき、私は、火曜日だから外来が大変だったのではないかと話しかけた。ところが、その場にいた全員が、私の顔をうかがったまま無言である。何かがおかしかった。後輩はようやく私に答えた。

「今日は金曜日ですよ」

私は凍りついた。曜日を間違えるなど普通ではあり得ない。

あり、本来は絶対に避けるべきである。実際、きちんと治療を受けていれば、私の症状はもっと早く良くなった可能性が高いと思う。

自分にとっては、まさに今この時、「現在」がスポットライトのように存在しているだけで、すでに、過去も未来も消滅していたのだということに突然気づいた。今日の曜日も、日付も、何年の何月であるのかも意味をなしていなかった。
　二人のナースは私に仕事を続けて欲しいと言ってくれたが、私は上の空で、レストランで座って話をしながら、食事を続けることが途方もなく苦痛に思われた。帰宅後、私は部屋の中に立ち尽くしたまま、認知症を発症したのではないかという恐怖に打ちのめされていた。
　うつ病では、自分が重大な身体の病気になったのではないかという心配が生じることがある。逆に言うと、うつ病には身体的な症状がつきものだ。食欲の低下、頭痛、便秘、口の乾き、動悸、疲れやすさ、その他いろいろな症状がみられる。そのため、最初はうつ病であることに気づかず、内科などの他の診療科を何カ所も受診してから精神科に紹介されるケースもある。心と身体は密接に結びついている。うつ病は決して気分や意欲だけの障害ではない。

7 うつ病の認識

精神疾患の患者さんは、自分が精神的に不調であることを認識できないことが多い。うつ病も例外ではない。自分が病気であることを理解することを病識というが、私が明確にうつ病であるという病識をもったのは、退職して数カ月たってからであった。

退職はしたものの、在職中にこなせなかった仕事や依頼原稿が山積みしていた。また、完全に仕事を辞めてしまえるほど蓄えがあるわけでもなかった。さらに、一度仕事を辞めたら二度と働けなくなるのではないか、という恐怖もあった。競馬に出走する競走馬と同じで、ゴールしたからといってその場で急停止することができない。退職した医療機関とは別の数カ所で、結局、パートタイムで週に四日働くことにしてしまった。

まず、締め切り期日の迫っている依頼原稿を書かなければならなかった。与えられたテーマで総説を書くには、関連する論文を少なくとも百ぐらいは読まなければならない。ただし、原著論文は執筆の形式が決まっており、緒言、研究対象、方法、結果、考察の順番で書かれ

ているので、慣れてしまえば読むのは難しくない。さらに、冒頭には抄録といって、全体の要約が短く記載されている。

ところが、論文のプリントアウトの山の前に座って最初の論文を手にとっても、読もうという意欲も興味もわいてこない。無理に読み始めると数行読んだだけでいやになってしまい、その先を読み続けることができない。ほんの短い抄録すら全部読むことができず、おまけに何が書いてあるのか、すぐにわからなくなってしまうので、同じ行を何度も読み返さなければならない。全く頭が働いていない感じである。

総説の締め切りはとっくに過ぎているのだが、何も書けないので二週間ほどすべての作業を放棄してしまった。その間にも時間はどんどん過ぎていき、いつも目の前にはまだ読んでいない山のような参考文献と、題名しか書かれていない真っ白なパソコンの画面が厳然と存在していた。

何とか仕事を進めようと悪戦苦闘しているうちに、あることに気づいた。朝は全く意欲がなくて、文献の題名を見て内容を分類することさえできないが、午後一時過ぎぐらいになると少し論文が読めるようになってくる。うつ病では症状に日内変動があることが知られてお

り、午前中に症状が重く、午後から夕方になると少し気分が楽になることが多い。もちろん、一日中同じように具合が悪い人もいるし、夕方のほうがつらいという人もいるが、午前中の具合の悪さはうつ病に特徴的な症状である。意欲や集中力が午後から多少改善するということに気づいたとき、私はそれがうつ病の特徴であることに、今さらながら愕然とした。

退職しなければならないほど症状が悪くなっていたことを、改めて実感した。そして日常生活の支障は、退職してパートタイムの仕事しかしていないにもかかわらず、依然として続いていた。これはただ単に一時的に気持ちが沈む、うつ「状態」ではなく、うつ「病」であることは明らかだった。そして、もうこれ以上、うつ病でないと自分を偽り続けることはできないことを悟った。

8　気持ちの沈み

午前中の意欲のなさに加えて、他にも、「そういえば……うつ病の症状ではないか」と思

い当たることがいくつもあった。うつ病の最も中核的な症状は気分の落ち込み、すなわち医学用語でいうと抑うつ気分である。ところがうつ病の人には、抑うつ気分を自覚していない人が案外多い。外来で診察していても、明らかに元気がなくつらそうな表情で、時によっては涙を流しているのに、「気持ちはそんなに沈んでいません」と言う人がいる。抑うつ気分よりも、不安やイライラ感を強く感じる人もいる。また、ひと言で抑うつ気分と言っても、その内容はさまざまであり、「元気がない」「何も楽しくない」「悲観的な感じ」「先がないような感じ」「絶望的な感じ」「泣きたい感じ」などいろいろな言葉で表現される。

ピュリッァー賞を受賞した新聞記者であり、のちに作家となったウィリアム・スタイロンは、自身がうつ病になり、精神病院で入院治療を受けた経験がある。彼はうつ病の闘病経験を『見える暗闇』という本の中に書いており、うつ病について「絶望を超えた絶望」であると表現している。気分が落ち込んだことがない人はいないだろうが、健康な人が日常生活上経験する抑うつ気分とうつ病の人の抑うつ気分は、程度も内容も全くと言ってよいぐらい違うものである。

たとえば、朝目覚めた瞬間に、不安とも悲しみともつかない何ともいえない気分の悪さがある。これからまた一日をやり過ごさなければならないが、そんなことに耐えられるだろうか。なんで目が覚めてしまったのだろうと思う。仕事のある日はやっとのことで顔を洗い、シャワーを浴びて家を出る。駅まで歩いていく途中で、いきなり、理由もなく涙が出そうになる。実際に泣くわけではないが、涙が込み上げてくるときの、あの胸の詰まるような感じがすることもあるし、実際に胸の痛みを感じることもある。窒息しそうな気がする。ようやく一回をやりすごしても、くり返し襲ってくるので、とにかく苦痛だ。相当な努力をしないと、歩いている最中に本当に涙が出てきそうであった。空気さえもが重く、呼吸をするのにもエネルギーが必要な感じであった。

うつ病評価尺度の一つには、面接の中に、「泣く」「涙ながらに話す」という項目がある。以前の私は、この項目の記載について、半信半疑であった。うつ病になったら泣きたいような気持ちになるかもしれないが、大の大人が「泣く」などということがあるだろうか。しかし自分が体験すると、やはりこの項目は現実の症状を的確にとらえていることに否応なく気

9 悲観

づかされたのであった。

意味もなく突然泣きたくなるという症状とともに、私の考えはだんだん悲観的になってきた。なぜ自分は能力もないのに精神科医になどになってしまったのか。二度と仕事ができないのではないか、経済的に生活できなくなるのではないか、という現実的な心配が頭をもたげてきた。

自分を責める気持ちは過去のことや抽象的なことにも及ぶようになった。いったい自分は何のために生きてきたのか、生きてきたこと自体が時間とエネルギーの無駄だったのではないか、これまでの自分の人生における選択はすべて誤っていたのではないか、家族にとっても自分は生まれてこないほうが幸せだったのではないか、もう何もかも取り返しがつかないと考えてしまう。

世の中には貧困や紛争に悩まされている地域がいくらでもあり、毎日多くの命が失われているというのに、恵まれた境遇にある自分が、こんな、ふがいない状況で生きていてよいのだろうか。誰か私の残りの命が欲しいという人があれば、身代わりにでもなりたいと思った。

これから先、何一つやりたいこともない、何一つ希望がない。

普段元気なときであれば、いちいち考えないようなことばかりが、ひっきりなしに頭の中をかけめぐった。それは本当にもう、どうすることもできない感じであった。

人は一つでも目標や希望があれば生きていくことができる。しかし、それがすべてなくなってしまったら……、これが「絶望を超えた絶望」ということなのだろうかと思った。

10　自殺

二人目の友人が亡くなった数日後に酒井先生から電話があり、私が自殺でもするのではないかということでみんなが心配していると言われた。なぜ自殺すると思われているのだろう

と私は不思議に思った。実際、そのときはどうしてもしなければならないことがあった。また、このような事態を想定してのことではなかったが、友人から「自分が死んだらこうしてほしい」と何度か言われていたことがあって、それをどのようにこなしていくかで頭がいっぱいだった。

友人の願いごとは簡単にできることではなく、準備に数ヵ月かかり、実行するのにも友人と生前親しかった人たちの助けが必要であった。そして、それを終えたあと、私の気持ちは急に落ち着かなくなってきた。

本当に危機的な状況になったのは、初夏の頃のことである。妙にそわそわジリジリして、家の中にいられなくなった。横になっても眠れない。時間をつぶしたいが、集中力がないために、趣味である読書もできない。そこで、街の中を何時間も歩き回るようになった。すると、翌日は疲れて起き上がれなくなった。

その次は、家中から不要なものや私的なものを、次々に処分し始めた。それは相当な量になった。処分するのにかなり躊躇するものもあったが、自分にもしものことがあったら何も残しておきたくないという気持ちが、思い出の品を身近におきたいという気持ちに打ち勝っ

た。そして処分してから、やはりこれでよかったのだと思うのだった。おかげで家からはすべての個人的な手紙や写真がなくなった。

私の趣味には、読書の他にダイビングがある。ダイバーにとってとても大切なログブックさえも、シュレッダーの中で細かく裁断された紙くずと化した。ログブックは文字どおり、ダイビングの記録である。ダイビングの日時、場所、サイト、ダイビング前後のタンクの空気圧、水温、最大深度、平均深度、透明度、ダイビングで見た生物や、一緒に潜ったダイバーからのコメントなど、自分のダイビングの歴史そのものである。ログブックは最後まで処分するのがためらわれた。しかし、最後の書きかけの一冊以外は破棄した。

そして、不眠がひどくなった。寝付きがとても悪く、開けた窓から夜のしじまに電車の音が聞こえてくる。夜の電車の音は、断続的に何時間も意識の中に入り込んできて、とうとうそれが途絶えると、終電車が通過したことがわかるのだった。そしてようやく眠りが訪れたかと思うと、数時間でいきなり覚醒する。午前二時か三時頃である。異様にはっきりした目覚めであり、一度目覚めると焦燥感が次第に強くなり、横になっていることができない。

そういう状態が何日か続いたあと、ある深夜、目覚めた途端に、いつもよりひどい焦燥感が襲ってきた。起き上がって、居間に行って明かりを点け、しばらくソファーに座っていた。

もう我慢できないと思った。キッチンに行って常備薬の引き出しを開けて薬の錠数を確認した。そして、ソファーに戻ってまたしばらく座っていた。

すると、ベッドで寝ていた猫がやってきてソファーに飛び乗り、私の隣に座った。猫はじっと私の顔を見上げていた。私も猫を見た。黒と銀色の縞模様の美しい毛並みで、透けるような緑色の目をしている。

猫はじっと私を見ている。私も猫の目を見ていた。猫にとって、目を直視されるのは相手からの攻撃のサインである。それなのに、猫は目をそらさずに私の顔を見続けている。その表情にも姿勢にも緊張や威嚇の徴はない。私は猫の頭を撫でた。ふわふわした柔らかい毛並みである。猫はまた、私の顔を見上げた。そのまま、ずっと見上げ続けている。

どれくらいたったのだろう。それはとても長い時間に思えた。

私はとうとう、「大丈夫だから」とつぶやいた。低くかすれて、自分の声ではないように聞こえた。

とにかく、死ぬのは明日まで待とうと思った。死ぬにしても、この家の中で自殺するわけにはいかない。猫に私の死ぬところを見せるわけにはいかない。猫のもらい手を決めてからでなければ、と思った。私が立ち上がってベッドに戻るまで、猫はソファーで横に座っていた。

実際に死ぬ手段を考えたことは何度かあった。しかしこのときは、実行したいという強い誘惑に駆られた。実行しそうになったのはその一度だけだったが、死にたい気持ちは、時によって程度が変化するものの、症状が重い間、常に続いていた。私は何とか、その気持ちを客観的にやり過ごそうとした。

死にたいという気持ちがわき起こること自体を、自分の意志で止めることはできない。それは自然にわき上がってくるからである。あるときには忍び寄るように、あるときは突然、晴天の霹靂のように強く。しかし、そのような気持ちが起きたとき、それはそれとして、原因はうつ病であるから普段の自分の考えとは違うのだ、と思うように努めた。少し離れた高いところから客観的に自分を観察しようとした。そうすると激しい感情の渦の底に引きずり

込まれそうな恐怖は多少和らいだ。

11　判断の誤り

うつ病では、ものごとの判断が難しくなる。判断するのに時間がかかるし、一度決めたあとでも、それが誤っていたのではないかと延々と悩む。普段とは異なる精神状態で、思考も悲観的であるから、大切なことを決定してはいけない。生死、結婚、離婚、退職、転居などは、うつ病が良くなってから考えないと後悔することになる。

退職は仕事上の理由があったので、私の場合はうつ病であろうがなかろうが退職することに変わりはなかった。退職は別にして、私もうつ病の判断力の低下のために、いくつかの大きな選択の過ちを犯した。

一つは、新しい仕事を始めようとしたことである。そんなことが始められる状態ではなかったにもかかわらず。いろいろな経緯があり、実行にいたる直前で計画は中止になった。そ

のために大変な迷惑をかけてしまった人もいて、自分が情けなかった。

　もう一つは宗教の勧誘である。私自身は特別な宗教を信仰していない。私の苦境を知ったある友人は、私のために信者が祈っていると言ってくれた。特別な助けが必要な人々のために、名前をあげて他の信者が祈りを捧げるのだそうだ。多数の中の一人であるとはいえ、信者でさえない、見ず知らずの私のために人々が祈りを捧げてくれたのだった。次に、その友人に会ったとき、私は入信を勧められた。普段であれば信仰についての自分の考え方をきちんと説明できたかもしれない。しかしそのときは、うつ病の経過が長くなってきたこともあり、この苦しさを取り除くためなら何でもしたいという藁をもすがる気持ちであり、曖昧な返事をしてしまった。

　しかし、信仰の問題は個人の人生観の根源に関わることであり、難しい問題である。私は、一カ月以上にわたって、入信するかどうかを考え続けた。

　結局、友人の属する宗教の信者にはなれないというのが結論であった。死にたいと思うほど症状が重くても、宗教に対する心の持ちようは変わらなかった。短い付き合いではなかったその友人に、自分の決断を伝えるのはとても気まずかった。友人をがっかりさせてしまっ

かなり悪化した。

たこと、それをきっかけに友情に軋轢が生じてしまい、もはや修復できなくなったこと、なぜ最初にもっと毅然と断らなかったのかと、自分を責めた。入信するかどうかという難しい問題についての決断を迫られ、また新たな人間関係のストレスにさらされて、症状はその後かなり悪化した。

ほぼ時を同じくして、別の宗教の信者からも入信を勧められた。ある医療機関に勤務している人から私が退職したことを聞いて、心配になったのだそうだ。しかし、私のことを話したという人間と私の間には何の付き合いもなかった。名前も知らなければ、言葉を交わしたこともない。

いずれの宗教の信者からも、早く入信を決断しないと苦痛が続いて危険だと言われた。それは症状や絶望感になおいっそう私の注意を向けさせることになった。私自身としては症状に巻き込まれるのを防ぐために、一歩離れて客観的に自分の状態を捉えようと努力している、まさにその時に。

偶然とはいえ、このような方法での複数の宗教への入信の勧誘は、他人に対する不信感と

恐怖をいやが上にも煽った。信仰をもたない友人が苦境に陥ったとき、信仰によってその人が救われるはずだと思って、善意から入信を勧めることがあるのだろう。しかし、前にも書いたように、信仰とは人の生き方に関わる問題であり、少なくともうつ病の経過中に入信するかどうかを考えるべきではないと思う。宗教の勧誘の他にもいろいろなことを勧める人がいるかもしれないが、それを試すよりも、まず休養して治療を受けることが大切である。

12 断酒

前に書いたように、私はいくつかの判断を誤ったが、幸運にもうつ病の改善を助けると思われることも決めることができた。それは断酒である。飲酒の習慣のある人は、うつ病になると飲酒量が増えることが多い。アルコールは少量であれば、緊張や不安をやわらげ、気分を多少高揚させる。そこで、アルコールを飲むと少し楽になったような気がして、どんどん酒量が増えてしまうことがある。なかには午前中から飲酒して、アルコール乱用にまで至る

こともある。

しかし、飲酒量が多くなりすぎると睡眠が浅くなる。二日酔いで体調も悪くなるため、ますます疲労感が強まる。飲酒してしまったことで自分を責める気持ちも強くなる。アルコールを飲み始めるときは、つらい現実から逃れられるように思うが、それはあくまで幻想であり、現実は何一つ変わらない。それどころか、うつ病のうえにアルコール性肝障害も背負い込みかねない。

私は十年以上にわたって晩酌の習慣があり、この間、飲まずに過ごしたことは数日しかない。どんな種類のアルコールも飲めるが、シャンパンやビールなど発泡性のものは大好きである。その私が断酒を決意したのは、偶然にいくつかの事情が重なったことによる。そのうちで一番大きな理由は、自分がうつ病であると認識してから飲酒量が増えて、アルコールの問題を抱えることが怖かったからである。実際、ほんのわずかでもリラックスできるのであれば、いくらでも飲みたかった。退職して仕事も減らしたため、二日酔いになっても当日休むこともできなくはない。しかし、そのことがかえって怖かった。

短くはない臨床経験上、アルコール乱用や依存の治療がいかに大変であるかということは、いやというほどわかっていた。また、患者さんは気づいていないだろうが、アルコールによる人格の変化は、いつも私を戦慄させた。

アルコールは節酒、すなわち飲む量を調節することがとても難しい。うつ病であればなおさらである。本当にアルコールによる障害を避けたければ、断酒するしかない。私は日常生活に何か問題を起こすような飲み方をしたことはなかったので、断酒する必要はなかったかもしれないが、この機会にアルコールをやめようと思った。毎日の飲酒量はたいしたことはなかったが、なにしろ飲酒歴が長いので、断酒後の数日間は禁断症状が出たらどうしようかと不安だった。しかし、幸いなことにそんな症状は一つも出なかった。ただ、なけなしの集中力を使い果たしてやっとのことで仕事を終えたあとなどは、無性にアルコールを口にしたくなることがあった。そういうときは、とりあえずその日は飲まずに翌日まで待って、それでもどうしても飲みたかったらまた考えようと思った。また、私が飲酒をやめたことを知ったT氏は、断酒が継続できるように、折に触れて励ましてくれた。

うつ病になったからといって、必ず飲酒をやめなければならないわけではない。しかし、もし飲酒量がどんどん増えるようであれば注意が必要である。

13　ジェットコースター

うつ病では、経過が良好であっても、途中で症状に波がみられるのが普通である。人間の身体は機械のようにはできていない。例えば、過労をきっかけとしてうつ病が発症した場合、休職したからといってすぐに症状が良くなり始めるわけではない。照明のスイッチをオンにしたり、オフにしたりするように、何月何日から具合が良くなったとか悪くなったとかわかる人もいるが、そういう人は躁状態を経験するような内因性、言いかえれば、より生物学的な障害の要因の強い人であり、そう多くはない。

うつ病では最も症状の重い時期を過ぎると、三寒四温といわれるように、症状が軽くなる過程で、一時的に悪化したように思えるときもある。このような症状の変動は、あらかじめ知らされていてもとてもつらいものである。実際、三寒四温などという生やさしいものではなく、症状が良くなったり、悪くなったり、激しい嵐の中にいるような感じがする。前に紹介したウィリアム・スタイロンも「うつ病（depression）」という英語は、この病気を適切に表現していないと書いている。脳の中で感情が嵐のように荒れ狂っているとしか言いようのない、うつ病の症状の激しさがデプレッションという言葉で弱められているというのだ。多

少おどけてはいるが「ブレイン・ストーム（brain storm）」とでも表現したほうがまだわかりやすいと言っており、私もそのとおりだと思う。

嵐の夜、森の中の迷路をあてどなくさまようイメージとでもいうべきだろうか。時々、大音響で落雷がある。とても寒く、暗い。大木の蔭に身を縮めても、冷たい雨が容赦なく背中を伝う。道がなく、どこを歩けば開けたところに出るのかわからない。移動しても消耗するだけだから、じっとしていたほうがよいのではないかと思う。しかし、何かに襲われそうな恐怖で動きたくなってしまう。叫びそうになる。
そして、なぜか、いつまで待っても夜は明けない。

イライラ感（焦燥感）のとても強い患者さんを何人も治療してきた私でさえ、自分がうつ病の経過中に、これほどひどい、まさに嵐の海で高波に翻弄されるような目にあわなければならないとは、思いもしなかった。
また、うつ病では経過中に正反対の症状が間隔をおいて出てくることがあり、これがまた、患者さんを疲労させたり不安にさせたりする。睡眠にしても、不眠が続いてひどく苦しい思

いをするときがあると思うと、一日のうち十六時間以上も眠ってしまうことがある。不眠と過眠である。普通は不眠が現れることが多いが、過眠になる人もいれば、両方を経験する人もいる。

食欲についても同じである。普通は食欲不振で食べられなくなり体重が減少する人が多い。一方で、逆に過食になったり、ペストリーやアイスクリーム、チョコレート、スナック菓子など甘いものが異常に食べたくなったりする人もいる。うつ病が悪化するときは食欲低下による体重減少があり、症状が改善してくると食欲が出てきて体重は元に戻る。しかし、そのような自然な形ではなく、食べるにしろ、食べないにしろ、食事の量が自分の意志でコントロールできなくなることがあるのだ。

私も同様の体験をした。一カ月ほどの間に五キログラムほど体重が減少してしまい、その後数カ月たってから異常な食欲の亢進が起こった。それは非常につらいことであったが、食事については放っておくことにした。無理に食事量のコントロールまで始めたら、ストレスが増すばかりである。結局、放っておいたのがよかったのか、やがて食欲の亢進は止まり、再び体重は多少減少した。

うつ病では、学業、家事、仕事などが日常生活に支障をきたすほどできなくなり、そのことについて患者さんは自分を責める。自分に甘えているのだと家族や周囲から責められることさえある。しかし、やりたくても気力がなくて何もできない。だから、うつ病の患者さんを励ましてはいけない。励まされると、彼らはもうどこにも行き場がなくなってしまう。

また、具合が悪くて自分の役割を果たせないことを常に気に病んでいるため、少し症状が軽くなると、これで回復の波に乗ったのだと早合点し、たまっている仕事をこなそうとする。あるいは、どこまで役割が果たせるか自分を試してみてしまう。私は常々うつ病の患者さんに、自分ができると思うことの半分だけやるようにアドバイスしているが、自分のこととなると、全く正確な判断ができなくなった。少し意欲が出ると、これでついに回復に近づいた、もう大丈夫だと思って、思いっきり仕事をしてしまった。結果は言わずもがなであり、その後は数日間、疲労感で起き上がることもできない。不安感やイライラ感とともに、まだ治っていないのか、という怒りがわき上がってくる。いったいいつまで、こんな状態を我慢しなければならないのか。

このようなときには、焦ってはいけない。焦るとよけいに感情の波に翻弄されてしまう。

時期が来ればうつ病は必ず治るのだから、とにかく待つことが大切である、時間がたつのを待つことが。そして、時間は決して止まらない。

14 たどりつけない迷路の出口

退職してから私は何度かパラオにダイビングに出かけた。ダイビングをしない人にとってはパラオといってもよくわからないかもしれない。太平洋西域のミクロネシアに位置する三百四十以上の島からなる共和国である。グアムから飛行機で一時間半ほどの距離である。

私とダイビングとの出会いは一種、運命的であった。親しい友人の島田氏の度重なる勧めで始めたのであるが、私はCカードとよばれるライセンスを一回で取得できなかった。そのときのライセンスコースのインストラクターは、資格をとったばかりの二十代の女性であった。海洋実習中に沿岸流にはまってしまい、インストラクターと私は漂流した。幸運にも海岸で私たちを見ていた他の二名の男性インストラクターがレスキューに来てくれたおかげ

で、海岸に戻ることができたが、そのときは恐怖のあまりコースを続けることができなくなってしまった。しかし、私はどうしても納得できず、他のダイビングショップを探して事情を説明し、最初から講習を受け直してライセンスを取得した。

ライセンス取得に再挑戦しようとしていた最中のことである。最初にショップに出かけたとき、そして、次にプール講習を受けた帰りにタクシーに乗ったのであるが、なんとドライバーが二人ともかつてダイビングをしていた。信じられないような偶然だ。そして二人とも、ぜひライセンスをとってダイビングを始めるように勧めてくれた。特に職業ダイバーであったという人は、「ダイビングは人生を変える、あなたの人生も変わると思いますよ」と言ってくれた。世の中に、そうそう人生を変えるほどのものがあるとは思えないので、私は俄然やる気になった。運動能力が皆無の私はダイビングの技術を習得するのにも人の何倍もの時間がかかったが、百本（タンクの本数で潜水の回数を数える）を超えたあたりから、海の中を少しずつ楽しめるようになってきた。

私たちは地上で重力の影響を受け、空気を呼吸して生きている。人工物に囲まれて。しかし、水中では地面を歩かなくてよい。BCDとよばれるジャケットにタンクの空気を出し入

れすることで、あるいは自分の呼吸を調節するだけで、垂直方向に好きなように移動できる。そして場所を選べば、人工物はいっさいない本当の自然と野生の海中生物に出会うことができる。ただし、タンクの空気がなければ海面まで生きては帰れないし、潮の流れが強いこともあり、ダイビングは厳しい自然の中に入っていくリスクをそれなりに伴っている。

色とりどりの美しい珊瑚礁の魚たち、優雅にひれをはためかせて飛んでいくマンタやイーグルレイ、数百尾のバラクーダやジャックフィッシュの群れ。わずかに身体を湾曲させるだけで強い流れに逆らって移動するサメの群れ。それらは、日常のすべてを忘れさせてくれる。また、強い潮流の中を流されていくとき、生き物としての人間の弱さ、非力さを思い知る。地上での境遇、地位、財産、そんなものはすべてはぎとられ、ただのヒトとしての自分に出会う瞬間がくる。

確かに、ダイビングは私の人生観を変えた。また、ダイビングを通して親しくなった友人たちが、うつ病になった私を支え続けてくれた。

退職前に診断書を書いて、希望する抗うつ薬を処方してくださった酒井先生は、共通の友人である世良さんとともに私を食事に連れ出し、さらには一時的に環境を離れるために沖縄

にまで連れていってくださった。そして、折に触れて「絶対、死ぬなよ」と言ってくださった。一度、なぜそこまで親切にしてくださるのかと聞いたことがある。すると先生は、同じダイビング仲間だから、と答えられた。実際、先生とは二度、ダイビングをご一緒したことがあった。また、ダイビングの扉を開けてくれた島田氏と菅野氏も私を食事に連れ出したり、頻繁に電話をかけてくれたりした。当時、電話がとても怖かったが、彼らの声が留守番電話から聞こえてくると、受話器をとることができた。電話の途中でいきなり泣き出したりする私に電話をかけるのはさぞかし気が重かったにちがいないが、それでも彼らは根気よく接してくれた。それは荒波で溺れそうになったときに差し出された救命ブイだった。

私がダイビングを始めたのは、一人目の友人を失う二年ほど前のことであった。当時はうつ病のきざしもなかった。その後、精神的に不調をきたし始めた頃、ダイビングは大きなストレス解消法になっていた。学生時代からダイビングや素潜りの豊富な経験があった島田氏も、就職してしばらくダイビングから離れていたあと、過労から体調を崩したのをきっかけにしてダイビングを再開したそうである。

ところが、最初のうちストレス解消になり、あんなに楽しく思えたダイビングに出かけることさえ、苦痛になってきた。宿泊場所やダイビングショップの予約はするのだが、実際に出かける予定の日が近づいてきても、全然行きたい気持ちにならない。こんな状態でダイビングができるのだろうか、おっくうだからキャンセルしてしまおうかと、ぐずぐず前日まで考え続けた。結局は出かけるのだが、今度はダイビングに集中できない。

ダイビングではガイドがついてポイントを案内し、珍しい魚、マクロと呼ばれるとても小さな魚、その他の海中生物、巨大な魚の群れなどを見せてくれる。しかし、ガイドの指差すその先に何がいるのかを見ることさえ、私には面倒になってきた。そんなことはどうでもいいという感じだった。そのため、ログブックは数字の羅列で、コメントの欄は白紙の状態が続いた。日付と天気と気温だけが記載されていて、肝心なその日の出来事が書かれていない日記帳と同じである。

〇年〇月〇日
ダイブサイト　ブルーコーナー

ダイビング開始時間　一〇：〇三、終了時間　一一：〇九
最大深度　二三・八ｍ、平均深度　一二・五ｍ
水温　二八・二度
コメント　…………（白紙）

そのかわりに、私は海底の見えない海の下を見ていた。初心者のときには、底が見えない深い海が不安だった。ウォールといって壁伝いにダイビングするときは、下を見るのが怖くて、横のウォールだけを見ていた。その私が、底のないブルーウォーターを見続けた。

うつ病の症状が重かったとき、いつも私につきまとっていたイメージがいくつかある。その一つは深く暗い海である。暗い海の中にいる自分が、少しずつ、少しずつ、細かくバラバラになって、何千メートルもの深い海の底に向かって静かに落ちていくというものだ。中深相（mid-deep zone）と呼ばれる数百メートル以深の海はもはや光の届かない暗黒の世界である。その暗黒の中を、見えないほど小さく、まさに海の藻くずと化して落ちていくというものである。

そのイメージを確かめるように、私は下方をただじっと見ていた。目を凝らせば、昏い中深層を、崩壊しながらどこまでも落下していく自分が見えるにちがいないと思いながら。

ブルーウォーターは、ただ暗く底なしのように見えるときもある。またその一方で、海面から陽光が差し込んで青くキラキラ光るのが見えるときもある。青く見えるときは、ずっと見ていると距離感や透明度がわからなくなってくる。宇宙の果てまで続いているように感じるときもあるし、すぐ近くに青い壁があるように見えるときもある。

ダイビングに行くことで、私は環境を変え、いろいろな思いから逃れ、暗いうつ病の迷路の出口を何とか探そうとしていた。しかし、それは容易には見つからなかった。出口が見えそうに思えると、次の瞬間それが幻想であり、まだ暗黒の嵐の中で身を屈めている自分を見た。迷路に出口があることさえ、信じることができなくなりそうだった。

15　鯨をめぐる旅

何回目かにパラオを訪ねたとき、たまたま、同じボートにビデオグラファーのT氏が同乗していた。彼はナショナルジオグラフィックをはじめとした各国のテレビ局にフィルムを提供する優れたプロフェッショナルであり、素晴らしい感性の持ち主である。彼がゲストのビデオを撮影していたので、私もDVDを作成してもらった。

私は帰国してから、DVDを作成してもらったこと、ダイビングをご一緒できて楽しかったというお礼を伝えた。その返信を見て驚いてしまった。最初の手紙のやりとりの文末はBest regardsやWarm regardsなどが普通で、Be strongとは書かないのではないだろうか。T氏にプライベートなことは何一つ話していなかったが、私の知り合いのガイドから友人を亡くしたことを聞いていたらしい。

その次に会ったとき、私は自分の症状を彼に話した。それはプライベートなことを他人に話さない私としては異例のことであった。彼は真摯な人柄なので私の症状について誰にも話すことはないだろうということが、なぜか直感的に確信できたのだった。彼は心配して、退

職しているとはいえ、もう少し仕事に費やす時間と労力を減らしたらどうか、とアドバイスしてくれた。

帰国してしばらくした頃、パラオのある島で鯨が座礁した。ちょうどいいから、パラオが鯨の回遊経路とどのような位置関係にあるのか調べてくれないか、という連絡がＴ氏から来た。何か仕事以外のことに関心を向けたほうがいいと思うから、と言ってくれた。

精神医学と何の関係もない、世界最大のほ乳動物である鯨のことを調べるのは、何か心をそそられるものがあった。しかし、鯨について、私は全く何も知らなかった。そこで神田神保町の三省堂本店に行って、鯨についての本を何冊か買って調べてみた。鯨の分類はある程度のことがわかったが、肝心の回遊経路については不明だった。おまけに種類によって回遊するものとしないものがいる。そこで、もっと安直に、専門家に直接聞いてみるのが最も早いのではないかと思い、Ｗ博物館の学芸員の櫻井氏にアポイントメントをとり、押し掛けていって教えていただいた。

櫻井氏は高校生の頃、Ｃ・Ｗ・ニコル（C.W. Nicol）の『勇魚』（いさな）を読んで日本の

古式捕鯨に魅せられ、米国東海岸の博物館で研究され、帰国後にW博物館の学芸員になられた方である。そして、『勇魚』の舞台になった、まさにその町に一年間滞在した場所なのだ。さらにその町は、C・W・ニコルがかつて『勇魚』の執筆取材のため一年間滞在した場所なのだ。

櫻井氏は研究テーマについての話の後で「私は鯨の回遊経路の研究を専門にしているわけではないので、S博物館の山田先生に紹介状を書いてあげましょう」と言ってくださった。専門家でもない、いきなり尋ねてきた一介の素人にここまで親切にしていただき、私はしみじみと人の温かさを感じた。そして、時代を超えて鯨と人間が織りなす不思議な関係に魅せられていた。

家に帰ってから、早速古本屋に『勇魚』を注文した（この本は残念ながら英語版も日本語版も絶版であり、古本しか手に入れることができない）。『勇魚』は、鮫に片腕を奪われた鯨取りの若者を主人公にした古式捕鯨に携わる人々の物語と、幕末の動乱の時代とを絡み合わせた一大歴史絵巻である。櫻井氏のおかげで、私は久しぶりに読書ができた。本が読めるということは、私にとって本当にうれしいことであった。

一方、山田先生にもアポイントメントをとった。山田先生は穏やかな笑みを絶やさない方であった。その研究室は、私のあこがれの、フィールドワークを専門にしている生物学者の研究室そのものである。廊下は暗く、部屋は狭くて、足の踏み場もないほどの本と資料の山、そしてガラス瓶に入ったホルマリンづけの標本。そして若い研究者が熱心に先生と話をしていた。
門外漢の私はじっと部屋の入り口で立っていたが、先生は他の研究者と話の途中なのに、「どうぞ、どうぞ」と招き入れてくださった。ここでもいろいろと教えていただいたが、鯨の回遊経路については解明されていないことがあまりに多いということを改めて知った。先生は本に書いてある分布図はあまり信用しないように、本来ならそれは標識をつけた鯨がこの場所で発見されたという「点」であるはずで、とても「面」では表せないと話された。

山田先生は保管庫で、天井まで埋め尽くされた鯨類の骨格を見せてくださったあと、回遊経路についてもっと調べたいのなら、パラオの倉田先生に聞いてみてはどうかと、関係機関にその場で連絡してくださった。ここでもまた、身に余るご好意をいただくこととなった（それとも私の変人ぶりが、櫻井氏から実に正確に山田先生に伝えられたのだろうか）。

倉田先生は、海洋生物の研究者なら、たいていお世話になったことのある、とても高名な先生だということだった。人見知りの私は、

「倉田先生というのはどんな方ですか、怖くないですか」
としつこく尋ねた。山田先生は、
「仙人みたいな人ですよ」
とおっしゃったが、仙人というのは現実離れしていて、私の不安をさらに煽るだけに終わった。聞かないほうがよかったかもしれないと後悔した。

そして、鯨を巡る旅はパラオに始まり、日本に来て、再びパラオに戻ることになった。私はパラオに戻って、T氏に鯨をめぐる旅の経過を報告した。実際にはほとんど何もわかっていないのだが。それでもT氏は静かに私の話に耳を傾けてくれた。

数日後、倉田先生を訪ねた。先生は第二次世界大戦前、パラオの南洋庁水産講習所を卒業され、南洋庁水産試験場勤務中に招集されてアンガウルの戦いを経験された。第二次世界大戦中、パラオは激戦地となり、ペリリューの戦いとアンガウルの戦いを併せると、日米両軍の犠牲者は約一万五千人にものぼった。倉田先生は戦後、東京都水産試験場、小笠原水産試験センター長を歴任され、現在はパラオ在住である。

倉田先生は信じられないほど博学で頭脳明晰である。人間のスケールが、何と言ってよいか、人間を超えている感じである。だから仙人と呼ばれるのだろうか。そして優しい方である。私には想像もつかないが、壮絶な修羅場をくぐりぬけてきた人特有の静けさというか、強さ、普通とは違った優しさをもった方である。そういう意味で、T氏と倉田先生は共通したところがある。

倉田先生は初対面の人を緊張させない。人間関係の緊張など、すでに超越しているのである。私は理由をつけて、三回も先生のところにお邪魔してしまった。それも、いつも約束の日時とは全然違う時であった。最初に電話したとき、先生は、

「あと十分ぐらいで来るのね。今シャワーから出たばかりで、何も着てないからさ」

とおっしゃるので、

「先生が何も着ていらっしゃらなくても気にしませんが……」

と、とんでもないことを答えた。

倉田先生の話に引き込まれ、なおかつ先生とT氏の間に勝手に共通点を見いだした私は、ぜひ二人をお引き合わせしたいと思い、いろいろと理由をつけて、多忙なT氏の迷惑も顧み

ず、彼を先生のところへ引っ張っていった。私の手元にはお二人の写真があるが、やはり、どことなく雰囲気が似ているのである。

お会いする前はあんなに心配していた私であったが、倉田先生の包容力に甘え、どんどん態度が大きくなった。三回目の訪問では、もはや連絡もせず、勝手に事務所に上がり込んだ。先生は、

「ちょっと待ってね。今シャワーから出たところで、お化粧する時間もなくて」

とおっしゃった（蛇足であるが先生は男性である）。いつもなぜかこんな感じになってしまう。

海亀がご専門ということで亀の話をうかがったが、先生は現在失われつつあるパラオの古い伝統や歴史を記録に残すことにも腐心しておられる。ご自宅も事務所もやはり、本と資料そして標本に埋もれていた。どれも宝の山である。

コロール市内を案内していただいたあと、海軍墓地に連れていっていただき、墓碑や記念碑の来歴をうかがった。

「墓地は北側を向いているでしょう？　日本のほうを向いているんですよ」
と先生はおっしゃった。丘の斜面から見える海が印象的だった。その色は、普段よりほんの少し、淡い色にみえた。

16　信頼

日本に帰って来た途端、私はまた調子が悪くなった。一日休んだにもかかわらず、仕事から帰ったあとは寝込んでしまった。しかし、もう自分の体調はあまり気にならなくなってきた。まだ治りきっていないのだからしかたがない。完全に元のペースで仕事をすることはできないかもしれないが、それでもいずれはもっと良くなるのだ。それに、どうして今までどおりのペースで仕事をする必要があるのか。誰も、私にそれを強制していない。がむしゃらに働かなければ自分の存在価値がないと、自分勝手に思っていただけなのだ。
そして今はまだ暗闇の迷路で出口を探しているとしても、まだ希望がもてなくても、この世界には素晴らしい人たちが生きている。櫻井氏、山田先生、倉田先生やＴ氏のように、そ

17 ある日の朝

れぞれが夢をもって。その人たちの夢を垣間みることができるだけで、私は幸せに感じることができるようになった。

嵐のようなうつ病の症状に翻弄され、自分を責め、絶望し、もう治りそうもないと思っていたとき、T氏は「あなたが元気であると信じます」と文末に書いてくれた。そのとき、自分が元気であるとはとても思えなかったが、彼が大丈夫と言うからにはたぶん私は大丈夫なのだろうと信じることにした。自分が信じられないときは自分を助けてくれる人の言葉を信じようと思った。

人を信じるというのは、私にとって最も難しいことの一つであった。しかし、うつ病になったおかげで、何とかそれもできるようになりつつある。うつ病になることも何かの足しにはなるのだ。何かどころではない、とても大切なものを手に入れることができたのかもしれない。

症状が最もひどかったときよりもだいぶましになってきたとはいえ、私の状態はあいかわらず、良くなったり悪くなったりのくり返しだった。前にも書いたように、うつ病が改善するときには症状に波があり、一時的に調子が悪くなることもある。むしろ、それが改善途上の一般的な経過である。しかし、私の症状の波は、だんだん良くなる方向に行くのではなく、横ばい状態で、ほぼ同じところを上がったり下がったりしているだけのように感じられた。あと一歩というところで、効果が頭打ちになっている印象である。

そこで、抗うつ薬を増量してみることにした。薬物療法のところで触れたように、副作用のため最初に服用した抗うつ薬を増量できていなかった。その後、別の薬に変えていたが、やはりいまだに効果が十分期待できるほどの量は服用していなかった。最初の薬で増量したときに副作用で苦しい思いをした経験があるので、二番目の薬を増量するのもためらわれたが、このままではいつまでたっても改善は望めそうにない。量を増やして、もしまた副作用で服用できなくなったら、別の薬に変更すればよいだけのことである。抗うつ薬はたくさんある。

そう思うと多少気が楽になった。

恐る恐る増量したのだが、今回は副作用がひどくなるということもなく、服薬を継続する

ことができた。服薬量を倍にしたから副作用も二倍になるということはないが、そうかといって副作用に慣れるとか、副作用が消失するということになるのかも感じられないときもあれば、ひどく不快で副作用止めの薬を併用しなければならないこともあった。副作用はほとんど感じなくてすむようになった。

そして十日ぐらいたったときのこと、驚くべきことが起きた。それまでは毎日、朝目が覚めたときに、表現しようのない何とも言えない気分の悪さ、悲しみ、不安、焦燥感、疲労感が奇妙に入り交じった気分の悪さに悩まされていた。

それが、ある日の朝、普通に目が覚めたのだ。別に不安でもなく、悲しくもなく、イライラもなく、疲れてもいなかった。目が覚めた瞬間、あれ？と思ったのだが、いつもと比べて何が違うのか、自分でも最初はよくわからなかった。何しろ、寝起きである。ベッドの中で、

ぼんやり考えているうちに、はたと、気分が悪くないことに気づいた。ベッドからも普通に起き上がれたし、クローゼットの前で座り込むこともなかった。二本足で立って顔を洗うこともできた。それは、信じられないほどうれしいことであった。「朝、普通に目が覚めること」はこんなに幸せなことだったのだと、しみじみ思った。

その後、「普通の朝」を迎えることのできる日数が少しずつ増えていった。抗うつ薬を増量した効果が出始めたのだった。集中力もだんだん元に戻ってきた。

長年同じことをやっていると、原稿や仕事の内容から、それらにどれくらいの時間が必要かわかるようになってくる。この原稿なら三日とか、この仕事なら二時間とかでものを考えたり、物事を処理したりすることができるようになった。また、目覚めたときに気分が悪い日は、その日を何とかやり過ごすことしか考えられないが、「普通の朝」には、これとこれをやっておこうというように、その日のスケジュールが頭に浮かんでくるようになった。

具合の悪いときには、じりじりするので、場当たり的に頭に浮かんだことをする。それが、とうば意味もなく街の中を歩き回るか、ひたすら寝ているかのどちらかであった。

とう、計画を立てて、秩序だった行動ができるようになってきたのだ。

さらに、実際に行動する前にスケジュールの優先順位をじっくり考えるようになった。頭に浮かんだことをすべて実行すると、必ずオーバーワークになるので、疲れてきて面倒くさくなったときにやり残した予定を翌日にまわせるように、優先順位の高いことから片付けるように気をつけた。しかし、それでもまだ不十分である。実際に疲れてしまったら、エネルギーを取り戻すのに数日かかってしまうので、疲れる前に物事をやめたほうがよい。その日にこなそうとしたスケジュールの二つぐらいはあえてやらないようにした。

「治りかけは特に注意して、できると思うことの五〇％ぐらいでやめておいてください」といつも患者さんに言っているこの私であるが、この「エネルギーをセーブする」ということがいかに難しいかが身にしみてわかった。かなり状態が良くなってこないと、秩序立てていてものを考えることもできない。力加減というものが実感できないので、自分の状態に合わせて仕事量をコントロールすることさえ難しい。

あるうつ病の患者さんが、だいぶ良くなってきたときのエピソードである。それまでは順調な経過だった。しかし、ある受診日に会ったとき、週の前半はよかったが、後半になって

疲れて寝込んでしまったということであった。彼は過労でうつ病になった。治療を始めた当初は疲労感が強くて、一日のうちで起きていられる時間がほとんどないほどであった。それが、治療が進むにつれてだんだん起床している時間が長くなってきていた。それなのに、どうしていきなり調子が悪くなってしまったのだろうか。

何か、具合の悪くなるようなきっかけがあったのかと尋ねると、週の始めの頃、一日四時間歩いたのだという。もともとウォーキングの好きな人なのだが、うつ病のために歩くことができなかった。気分が良くなってきたから運動不足の解消もかねて歩いたのだという。

私はびっくりしてしまった。元気なときでさえ、四時間のウォーキングにはとてもついていけない。まして彼は数週間前までは、起き上がっている時間より寝ている時間のほうが長かったのである。

一日四時間歩いたら疲れて寝込むのは当然であり、うつ病が悪化したのではないこと、歩くのはかまわないが、せめて一時間ぐらいにして、疲れる前にやめておくように説明した。

これは極端な例だが、患者さんは良くなりかけるとつい安心して、目いっぱい活動してしまう。うつ病を順調に治すためには、できることもあえてしないという勇気が必要なのである。

朝起きたときに、その日のスケジュールが思い浮かぶようになると、午前中にも仕事をしたり、本を読んだりできるようになってきた。思考のスピードが遅くなる症状を「思考抑制」というが、思考抑制が改善する過程は、まるで停止している自動車にエンジンをかけて、サイドブレーキを解除して滑らかに走り出すときの感じに似ている。明らかに思考の速度が速くなってきたのがわかる（といっても以前に比べてという意味だが）。さらに、複雑なことや、込み入った仕事もこなせるようになってくる。何かを決断したあとも、決めたことが間違っていたのではないかとくよくよ考えることもない。

鏡を見ると、自分の表情がはっきりしてきたのがわかる。話す速度も声のトーンも変わってくる。具合の悪いときは、生気のない、ぼんやりした、影の薄い印象になる。イライラして怒りっぽく見える日もある。声も小さくなるし、話し方も遅くなる。

長年外来で診療に携わっていると、病歴の長い患者さんについては、診察室のドアを開けて部屋に入ってきた瞬間に、調子が良いか悪いかがわかるようになるものだ。それぐらい、外見からして違ってくるのである。

もちろん、調子の良い日ばかりが続くわけではない。時には、朝目覚めたときから調子が悪

い日もあるし、集中できないこともある。異常に眠かったり、だるかったりするときもある。
しかし、それはそれでいいか、と思えるようになった。確実に改善する方向に向かっているのが実感できるので、早めに横になって疲れをとるようになった。

18　笑う

うつ病になると、何一つ楽しいと思えなくなる。自分の趣味や、最も好きなことが楽しめなくなったら、うつ病の症状はかなり重いと思ってよい。したがって、その前の段階として、「趣味はなんとか楽しめるが仕事はできない」ということがうつ病ではあり得る。怠けているのではなくて、症状の程度の問題なのである。自分の一番好きなことさえ楽しくなくなると、もはや心の底から笑えなくなる。

外出して人と会うことができれば、言いかえれば、家で寝たきりになっていなければ、人前でにこやかな表情をつくることは可能かもしれない。しかし、それは調子の悪いところを人に見せまいとする努力の結果であって、楽しいことがあったからとか、うれしいことがあ

ったから、にこにこしているわけではない。「スマイリング・デプレッション」という言葉があるほどで、他人にはなんとか普段どおりの自分を見せようとしてしまうことが多い。

しかし、もはや自分の表情を取り繕うことができなくなると、誰にも会いたくなくなる。さらにひどくなると、人ごみや道で見ず知らずの人とすれ違うことさえ、圧迫感を感じて怖くなる。どこにも出かけたくなくなる。

「パーソナリティー」という言葉は、ギリシャ語の「ペルソナ」に由来することはよく知られている。ペルソナは「仮面」という意味であり、人は誰でも他人と一緒にいるときは、「他人に見せる自分」という仮面をかぶっている。うつ病では、仮面をつけることさえ重労働である。仮面をつけない自分はとても繊細なものであり、もし他人に傷つけられたら修復不可能であるような気がして、とても人前には出られない。

長い間、私は楽しくて、あるいは面白くて笑うということがなかった。笑うことなど、これから先ありそうもないと思うような日々であった。しかし、「普通の朝」が訪れるようになって、しばらくしてから、ふと本屋に行ってみようと思いついた。一週間に三回ぐらいは

書店に行く読書好きの私が、もう何週間も行きつけの書店に足を運んでいなかった。写真が多いダイビング雑誌さえ買う気になれないのがわかっていた。しかし、その日はなぜか、何か面白そうな本が読みたいと思った。

久しぶりに八雲堂書店で見慣れた配列の書棚の前に立つと、懐かしい気がした。集中力がないと書棚にずらりと並んだ本の題名を見ることさえおっくうなのだが、そのときは本の題名を追うことができた。そして、一冊の本が私の興味を引いた。それは、落語家である桂文珍が慶應義塾大学で講義をした内容をまとめた『落語的笑いのすすめ』であった。普段は何冊も本を買うのだが、その日はその一冊だけを買って家に帰った。

本を開いた。さすが落語家である。私はすぐに、数百人は収容できるはずの大きな講堂で、学生の一人として聴講しているような錯覚に陥った。場の作り方、聴衆の関心の惹き方、話の構成などがとにかくすばらしい。しかも、噺家として羽織を着て高座にすわっているのではなく、学生を相手に日本の伝統芸能について講義をしているのだ。さらに、講義の内容がとても面白かった。恥ずかしながら、落語を聞いたのはほんの幼いときで、それも一度か二度しかない。もちろん噺家の名前も内容も全然覚えていない。それなのに、何の知識のない

私でも、みるみるうちに引き込まれていって、決して飽きさせない。そして、笑いの連続である。思わず声を出して笑ってしまう。一気に文庫本一冊を読み切ってしまえそうだったが、長時間集中した翌日の疲労を思い出して、かろうじて読むのを我慢した。この本を読み終わってしまうと、楽しみがなくなって、そのあとが困ると思い、翌日、外出のついでに、何件か書店を巡って彼の本を探した。そして本を買いだめしてから、最初の一冊目を読み終えた。

今ではインターネットで何でも注文できる。本もネットで注文して、至急配送をクリックすれば翌日には手に入れることができる。しかし、それでは何か違う気がした。自分で書店に足を運び、ときには何件も回ってから自分の探していた本を見つける喜びは、読書好きにはたまらなくうれしいものである。この「書店巡り」もできるようになった。

こうして、私は再び本当に笑うことができた。そして、遅まきながら、自分がいつも診察中に気をつけていることを思い出した。それは、なるべく患者さんに診察室の中で笑ってもらうということである。精神科では長期間の通院が必要な人が多い。何年あるいは十数年に

わたって記載された分厚いカルテ（あまりに厚くて分冊になっているものもある）を見ると、長年病院にかかって、服薬するということはどんなにストレスだろうと思う。通院歴の長い人の場合、特に必要なければ私から症状についてきくことはしない。どうしても自分の状態について話したい患者さんは、世間話をしてでも、きちんと伝えてくれる。具合が悪くても口に出さずに我慢してしまう私の話の腰を折ってでも、きちんと伝えてくれる。具合が悪くても口に出さずに我慢してしまう人、症状を的確に教えてくれる人、大げさに気にしすぎる人、それぞれ長年の付き合いでわかってくる。

というわけで、病歴が長い人には通院のストレスを少しでも軽くするために、また、初めて受診した人には緊張や怒り、悲嘆を軽くしてもらうために、診察室の中で笑ってから帰ってもらおうというのが私のポリシーである。冗談やダジャレを言わなくても、人を笑わせることはできる。私自身が笑いのネタになっていることも多々ある。また、笑わせることができなくても、診察室の中で怒りをあらわにしたり泣き出したりした人をそのままの気分状態で帰してはいけないことは鉄則である。

精神科の診察室の中で涙を流す患者さんは少なからずいる。各診察ブースにはティッシュペーパーの箱が置いてあるが、それは医者が風邪を引いたときに使うためのものではない。

患者さんが涙を流し始めたときに、すかさず差し出せるように置いてあるものだと、常々私は思っている。そして、ティッシュペーパーの箱は、結構な頻度で活躍しているのだ。

人は心から笑うことができれば、その一瞬、心がすっとして浄化されたように感じる。『落語的笑いのすすめ』にも笑いの効用について書かれているが、楽しい、うれしい、面白いという感情を伴った笑いは、ヒトにとってとても大切だ。うつ病に関して言えば重症度のバロメーターにもなる。

心から笑った自分を見て、これでやれやれ一安心だ、と思った。何度か笑えるようになると、あたりがほんのわずか明るくなったような気がした。

迷路の出口から、光が差し込んできているのだ。

19　存在の支え

さて、ある程度以上の重症のうつ病の治療では、抗うつ薬の服用と休養が不可欠だという

ことは以前に書いた。しかし、それと同じくらい大切なのは、周囲からの支えである。通常、最初に思い浮かぶのは家族だろう。温かく見守ってくれる家族がいる患者さんは本当に幸運であると思う。

しかし、恵まれた状況ばかりとは限らない。家族がそばにいなかったり、一人暮らしであったりする場合もある。残念なことに、家族がうつ病に対して理解がなく、偏見をもっていることさえある。自分の家族の一人がうつ病だとは信じたくない、あるいは認められない人たちもいる。

たとえ家族がいなくても、理解がなくても、うつ病になったときに患者さんを支えてくれる人は必ず存在するものである。治療を開始すれば、治療者はもちろんサポートしてくれる。しかし、治療者と話ができるのは短時間であるから、なるべく多くの支えがあったほうがよい。もし、あなたがうつ病になったら、思いもかけない人たちが支えになってくれる可能性がある。それほど親しいと思っていなかった人、自分のことを心配してくれるとは思ってもみなかった人たちが助けになってくれることがある。だから、いつでも自分の心を開いていることが大切だ。

反対に、自分が助けてほしいと思う人、それまで親しく付き合っていると思っていた人たちが無関心で冷たい態度をとったり、距離をおいてよそよそしくなったりするという体験も私の場合にはあった。何度説明しても理解してもらえないこともあった。自己中心的な思惑から親切の押し売りのようなことをする人もいた。このような体験は、うつ病になって人間関係に敏感になり、恐怖さえ感じている私の苦痛にさらに追い討ちをかけた。

しかしかえって、そのようなつらいときだからこそ、誰が本当に自分を心配してくれているかがはっきりわかった。仕事ができなくなってしまった自分、気分がふさいで陰気になっている自分、くよくよして活気がない自分、イライラして怒りっぽい自分、精神的な不調に悩む自分をそのまま受け入れてくれる人たちがいた。その人たちは決して押し付けがましくなく、私を心配していることを伝えてくれた。時々連絡をくれたり、疲れない程度に会ってくれたりした。私は、その人たちが自分のことを心配してくれているということを感じているだけでよかった。そして症状がつらいときに、こんな自分でも心配してくれている人がいるのだということを思い出すと、それだけで安心できた。

20　エピローグ

以前、ある抗うつ薬のパンフレットが気に入って、しばらくデスクの前に貼っていたことがある。朝、白いバスローブを羽織った女性が歯磨きをしようとしている写真である。洗面

支えてくれる人が見つかるまでには、しばらく時間がかかるかもしれない。そのようなときには、人でなくてもよい。もしあなたが、犬や猫、その他の動物の世話人なら（飼い主なら）、彼らは立派なナーシング・アニマルになってくれる。

私の猫は、私がほとんど一日中ベッドから起き上がれなかった間、何時間でも付き添って、そばで寝てくれた（もちろん好意からそうしているわけではなくて、ただの習性であるが）。手を伸ばしてふわふわした温かくて柔らかい毛玉に触れると、ゴロゴロ喉を鳴らすくぐもった音が聞こえてきた。私が眠れない夜でも、静かな寝息が聞こえて、時々寝言も言っていた。

その他、写真でも本でも音楽でも、苦痛を和らげてくれるものは、探せば結構、身近に存在している。心を開いていると、おのずから心に訴えかけてくるものがわかる。

台の上には茶色のトラ猫が座って彼女の顔を見上げている。今にもゴロゴロ喉を鳴らす声が聞こえてきそうな満ち足りた表情の猫である。「晴れやかな朝に、さわやかな気分」というような意味のコピーがついていた。

そのときは何となく気に入っていただけだったが、うつ病を経験した今では、モーニング・デプレッションという「朝の症状の重さ」が改善したときの様子を的確に表現した、実によくできたパンフレットだったと思う。

平和な朝である。

毎日というわけにはいかないが、たいがい、私も普通の朝を迎えられるようになった。偶然の一致だが、私が歯磨きをするときも猫が洗面台の上に飛び乗って、額を私の身体にこすりつける。正式な朝の挨拶は額と額をくっつけ合うものだと思っているらしく、猫は私が身を屈めるまで、洗面台の上を行ったり来たりして注意を引こうとする。

そして私は再び、ダイビングを楽しむことができるようになった。意味もなくブルーウォーターを見続けることはもはやなくなった。T氏とダイビングするときは、彼の邪魔になら

ないように一人で自分のダイビングを楽しむことができる。そして、海の中でのコミュニケーションに言葉は必要ない。言葉を超えた直接的で瞬時のコミュニケーションが可能である。このようなコミュニケーションのありようと心地よい感覚は、それこそ言葉にするのが難しいのだが。

ログブックには、魚、カメ、マンタ、その他、海で出会った生き物たちのイラストがまた登場するようになった。イラストに色を塗り、図鑑で名前を調べて書き写すことができるようになった。

とりわけ印象に残っているのは、傷を負いながらも生き延びている個体だ。右の後肢がちぎれたカメ、尾が折れて山形に変形したイーグルレイ、尾が付け根からちぎれたマンタ。捕食者に襲われたのだろうか。それでも彼らは危機を脱出し、生き延びた。山形に変形した尾をもつイーグルレイには、最初に出会ったダイブサイトとは別の場所で、また再会した。

とにかく、生き延びることが大切だ。じっと待っていれば、必ず新しい明日がやってくる。道を歩いて角を曲がると、全く別の風景が見えるときがくる。

思い返してみて、もう二度とうつ病にはなりたくないと思う。私の中で、決して元に戻らない、失われてしまった何かがある。さらに私は、うつ病が再発しやすい障害であることを知っている。一生のうち一度だけうつ病のエピソードを体験するのか、あるいは何回かくり返すのか、それは誰にもわからない。しかし、もし次のエピソードを体験しなければならないとしても、そのときの私はうつ病になる前の私とは違う。再発したときには、以前の経験が必ずエピソードを乗り越えるときの助けになるだろう。

そして、うつ病の苦痛を経験することによって、私は素晴らしい出会いを経験し、人の温かさを知った。今までとは別の生き方や考え方を身につけた。感謝すべきことではないだろうか。

反射光

マーク・ソープ

　四頭のコビレゴンドウが大きな群れから離れてまっすぐ私のほうへやってきた。鯨たちが近づくにつれ、彼らの発するソナーに反響して、私の胸腔が振動した。おかしな生き物に対する好奇心につられて、鯨たちが調べにやってきたのだ。十メートルの距離を一瞬にして通り過ぎたとき、彼らの敏捷さとスピードに私はただただ驚嘆していた。鯨たちの漆黒の瞳をじっと見つめると、彼らが理知的な動物であることがわかった。個体であれ群れであれ、もしも彼らがその気になったら、まさに今ここで自分の生命が終わりを遂げることも、私にはよくわかっていた。しかし、彼らはそうしなかった。その代わり、いつものように闖入者としてではあるけれども、私は彼らと「魔法の瞬間」を共有したのだった。水中の世界、それは人が普通に考える以上に、私にとっては特別に自分の家と感じられる場所である。

私は、イングランド南海岸にある公立の養護施設で育った。姉と私は、祖母や里親のもとでそれぞれの人生を踏み出した。どちらの道もうまくいっていなかった。祖母も里親もお手上げ状態になったため、私は養護施設に移った。そのときから、私の「家族」は私や姉と同じような境遇の数十人の子供たちになった。

　言うまでもなく、姉と私の関係は、普通の家庭環境の中で培われる親密さとは、悲しいほど遠くかけ離れたものであった。あまりに多くのことが起こりすぎているのだった。私たちはお互いを理解し認め合っていたが、ただ親密な関係を築くチャンスがなかった。孤独で自分だけが頼りであり、ごく幼いときから、自分には兄弟姉妹がいないのだと思うようになっていた。

　当時の英国の社会福祉制度のもとでは、軍隊に入隊することが、十六歳の私に残されたほとんど唯一の選択肢であった。もし十七歳になって仕事が見つけられなければ、この保護された環境から否応なく外に出され、自分で何とか生きていかなければならない、と言い渡され

ていたからだ。適性検査で充分な成果をあげるやいなや、私は入隊申請書にサインした。こうして、今回は自分の自由意思によるものとはいえ、私はまた別の「施設」に入ることになった。今日に比べて戦うべき戦争のさほど多くない保護的な環境は、現代社会で雑多な責任を負わなければならないという現実から、私を守ってくれた。私がそう思っている限りにおいて、軍隊は安全な場所であった。

一九八〇年代初頭、十八歳のときに歩兵連隊兵士としてベルファストで体験したことは、凄惨を極めた。この経験は、私が平和で平穏な環境を望むようになる長い過渡期のはじまりとなった。ゆっくりと自転する私たちの惑星の上で、自分たちが繰り広げている暴力や憎しみのない環境を求める転換点であった。どうしたら人間は、あのような邪悪な存在——爆破、強迫的な暗殺行為、仲間の殺戮をも正当化するような憎悪に満ちた存在——になれるのだろうか。ある人々がいかにして、お互いにこのような苦痛をもたらすことを正当化できるのかは、私の理解を超えていた。そのうえ、さらにひどいことに、その苦痛を充分理解しないうちに、そのまっ只なかに捕捉されてしまった。これは狂気だ。私は、暴動、爆撃、殺人、そしてさまざまな狂信的行為を目撃した。

軍隊で過ごした期間中ずっと、私は深酒し過ぎたあとの、酩酊としらふの間のような無感覚な状態であった。そしてある日目覚めたとき、私は自分が国家への忠誠を、いつの間にか生活の手段にすりかえていたことに気づいた。英国歩兵部隊を退役したら、次は、フランス語を話し、フランス外人部隊の燃え上がる手榴弾の徽章をつけ、各自それぞれに異なった理由で各国から入隊してきた兵士たちで成り立っている不可思議な部隊に従軍していた。仲間の兵士に従軍に至る経緯を聞くことは「不適切」であると見なされていたので、私もその暗黙の了解に基づいて、匿名性という安心できるシェルターを利用していた。ともに過ごした元英国軍兵士も何人かいたが、私たちはただ通常の「勤務時間」外に話をするために一緒にいるだけだった。

私は最初の任地として、アフリカ大陸先端のジブチで従軍した。第十三歩兵師団に二年間所属したが、この経験があったからこそ、今の私が存在している。転機はそのときに訪れた。

部隊のフランス兵の一人との雑談をきっかけに、私はたまたまダイビングを習うことになった。そして、ダイビングを通して、紅海の下に自分が自由になれる世界を発見した。それ

までの人生で経験したどんなこととも違う、素晴らしい体験であった。かつて子供の頃、自分がいつも自然に魅せられていたことを、私はまた思い出した。私たちは英国南部の森の近くに住んでいたので、勝手知った土地でいつも小川を飛び越え、イモリ探しに熱中していた。ジブチの穢れのない珊瑚礁でのダイビングは、理性と自由をもたらし、そして、希望を与えてくれた。私は軍隊生活の最後の年が終わるのを心待ちにし、それから、とうとう自分自身を見つける生涯の旅に向けて船出した。

この、逃げ場のない拘束状態と暗黒のストーリーを読むと、私には、友人が翻弄されたうつ病のときの気持ちが理解できる。私は自分が人生の中でうつ病になったことがあるとは思っていなかったが、それは個人がうつ病をどう認識するかによると思う。ある人は他の人よりもより耐久力が強い。私はうつ病になったことはないと思う。けれども、自分がうつ病になったかどうかが判断できるようなもの差しを今までもっていなかったので、過去にそうなったことがあったとしても知る由がなかった。しかし、私が除隊して別の人生を歩み始めた途端に、とても重い肩の荷が降りたことは明らかである。

私は過去のいくつかの出来事に暗黒を見るが、それらの暗黒があるからこそ、幸福の記憶

を呼び起こして私の「幸せの道」を思い描くことができる。そのルートは高いところ（幸福）もあれば低いところ（苦難）もあるが、幸運にして低いところより高いところのほうが多い。人の心には記憶を再構成する機能が備わっていると思う。たとえば私の子供時代のことを思い返すと、楽しくほのぼのとした思い出がある。それらの出来事を思い出すと、同じ時期に経験したつらい記憶を難なく修正することができる。「幸せの道」は記憶を再構成して幸福を実感する方法なのだと思う。

私は容易に幸福を感じることができる。なぜなら、飾り気のないものがより私に感動を与え、そして我が身一つでも満足だから。私には最新の流行の品は全く必要ないし、快適に過ごすためのあれやこれやも必要ない。シンプルな生き方が私には最も似合っている。

良くも悪くも、私が生きることの意味を判断する唯一の方法は、自分自身の人生経験であ
る。私は誰もがみな人として、合理的に考え、他人を愛し、純粋な人間性に感謝する能力をもっていると信じている。たとえ、ある人々はその他の人々より合理的な思考やヒューマニティーを感じるのにより多くの努力が必要だとしても。そのような能力は誰の中にも存在し、

日の目を見るのを待っている。私は波間の下に自分の幸福を見いだした。私は自分を感動させ、こんなにも長く愛してやまないダイビングをこれからも続けていくつもりだ。

私と著者との友情は、絶え間のない深い信頼と感謝によるものである。かつての誤解を、話し合い、理解することで乗り越え、今では期待と可能性が存在するようになったと信じている。これからも私は著者をサポートし、親友であり続けるつもりだ。

迷い込んだ不死鳥

倉田　洋二

　早朝のスコールに目を覚ます。ベランダに出て夜明けの空を仰ぐ。五時二十分。東の空が薄明るい。アマサギの群れがねぐらから餌場に向かう時間だ。一羽から二羽、時に四、五十羽、約三十分の間に百五十羽前後カウントできる。が、五月に入ってこの二日間、一羽も飛ばない。日本へ旅立ってしまったのだろう。パスポート不要の三千キロ自力飛翔の旅、ふとうらやましく思う（栄養失調で餓死した若い戦士の残された日記の中に、「この海の上を歩けるなら歩いても日本に帰りたい」とあった）。

　八時、南に目を向ける。緑の岩山、青い海、白尾熱帯鳥が一羽長い尾を引いて滑空している。見慣れたパラオの風景、だが私には至福のひとときであり、バードウォッチングの日課

の始まりである。ベニスズメ、オニメジロ、カラスモドキ、ナンヨウショウビン。鳴き声をキャッチするため、電話機の音も低くしてある。その静けさをそっと破るような呼び出し音に受話器を耳に当てると、短いP音。それは私と外地（パラオ以外）をつなげる期待の一瞬である。三千キロ彼方の日本から、電話の主の声が聞こえてくる。

数カ月前、私のフィールドオフィスに、この電話の主が侵入して来た。来意を告げられ、滞在中に数回パラオの鯨（くじら）類、儒良（ジュゴン）等その他、古き良き時代の熱帯生物研究所の奇人変人の大先生方のお話やパラオの原始生活のお話をした。二度目の来パの折、電話の主は一冊の原稿を私に下さり読んでくれと言う。斜めに目を通すと、うつ病にかかった本人の精神分析、うつ病の闇への航海──」とあった。見ると表紙に「普通の精神科医?──症状と治療過程、快癒までが明快な文章でつづられている。最後に気になる文章があった。それは過ぎる大戦で孤島で生き残った若い兵士（精神科医）との出会いとその交友の一部である。かつての若い兵士はヨタヨタの老兵で、日本を逃れ南海の島で海に山に自然と遊び、海洋生物学徒として見果てぬ夢を追っている。彼は「うつ病は文明病で海に山に三人に一人はいる。本人が気付かないだけ」と割り切っている。彼は医者嫌いで

もあるが、老いは好むと好まざるとにかかわらず、医者の世話になる今日この頃である。くだんの精神科医はこの老兵こそ探していた救世主だったと褒め称えているが、冗談ではない。精神科は医学の中でも最も難しい分野であろうと思う。正常とも異常とも思える患者の言語行動からその内に秘めたる精神状態をつぶさに洞察し、的確なる判断をして治療に当たらなければならない。外科医のように目に見える患部をバサバサ切断して治療するのとは全く異なるのである。

　私に会いに来た精神科医は探し求めていた奇人変人のカメ仙人をパラオの片隅から見つけ出し、その言語行動に浮世を忘れて共鳴し、挙句の果てに手放しで褒め称えている。この精神科医がカメ仙人の言語行動に共鳴しなくなった時こそ、うつ病が治ったときであろう。最初に会ったときから〇カ月、逢う毎に健康になって来たのが私には解る。どうか、パラオの自然にどっぷり浸かって不死鳥のようにたくましく甦ることを祈りたい。

あとがき

日本における自殺者数は一九九八年から年間三万人を超えており、交通事故死よりも多い。この背景には社会的要因をはじめとしていろいろな問題が考えられる。また、うつ病に対する一般の人々の認知度がまだ低く、治療を受けていないうつ病患者が存在すること、精神疾患や精神科医療に対する偏見なども影響していると考えられる。日本でも、専門家による一般向けの優れたうつ病の解説書が多く出版されている。今更、私がさらに一冊を加える必要はないのかもしれないが、本書が、うつ病に悩む当事者の方々をはじめとした多くの人たちのお役に立つことを願ってやまない。

本書の作成には共著者であるマーク・ソープ氏、翻訳者であるリー・ダンシー氏をはじめ多くの方々のお世話になった。私の体験した症状を記録に残しておくよう勧めてくださった酒井先生にも心から感謝申し上げたい。

「記録に残しておくといっても、とてもパソコンに向かって文章を書けるような集中力も

気力もありません」と訴える私に、それならテープレコーダーに吹き込んでおいてはどうかとまで言ってくださったのは酒井先生である。テープレコーダーは使用しなかったが、なるべく症状についてメモを取るように心がけた。そして記録する作業により、自分の症状に巻き込まれそうになりながらも、そこから一歩身を引いて、なるべく客観的に自分を観察しようと試みた。そのことは、症状の苦痛を緩和する大きな助けになったのである。

マーク・ソープ氏には写真をご提供いただいただけでなく、数々のアドバイスやサポートをいただいた。本書に書かれたことは、それらのほんの一部に過ぎない。「普通の精神科医?」という本書のユニークな題名も表紙のデザインも、彼のアイディアによるものである。彼の最新のフィルム「The Majesty of Muck」（泥濘のきらめき）は、二〇〇七年十月にアンティーブ（フランス）で開催された第三十四回国際水中映像フェスティバルにおいて、Prix du Public賞（ピープルズ・チョイス賞）を受賞した。

リー・ダンシー氏は、思考抑制といううつ病の症状の影響とはいえ、適切な表現が思いつかず意味をなしていないような私の文章を、精読して翻訳してくださった。とてもわかりづ

らかった当初の文章が出版にこぎ着けられるまでになったのは、膨大な時間をかけたダンシー氏とのディスカッションによるものであり、感謝の念に耐えない。自分で書いておきながら日本語の表現に納得できず、翻訳された英文をみてようやく、「そうそう。これが自分の言いたいことだった」と理解するということも度々であった。翻訳文から、本文の校正を行なったこともあった。

また、星和書店の石澤雄司社長や編集者の曽根裕子氏、デザイナーの高山由美子氏のご支援がなければ、この本は決して日の目をみることはなかった。石澤氏も曽根氏も多くを語られないが、うつ病に悩む多くの方々にささやかではあるがお役に立ちたいという私の気持ちを、真摯に受け止めてくださった。心より感謝申し上げたい。

二〇〇七年十月

明　海

翻訳者

リー・ダンシー

カリフォルニア大学バークレー校在学中に日本に興味をもつようになる。1988年に初来日後、フルタイムの翻訳者として活躍している。現在、妻と3人の子供たちとともに北海道に在住。

翻訳者からのメッセージ

『普通の精神科医？―うつ病の闇への航海―』を翻訳する前まで、私はうつ病に関連した本を読んだことがなかった。本書を読んで、うつ病について解りやすく書かれていることに驚きを禁じ得なかった。ちょうど幼なじみの友人から、その人の身に起こったことを聞かされたような感じだった。著者のダイビングや読書に対する愛着などの個人的な事柄は、一見するとうつ病と関係がないように感じられる。しかしこれらのエピソードは、人間としての著者を差しおいて疾患としての「うつ病」がこの本の中心になってしまうのを防いでいる。うつ病のことにだけにとどまらない日常生活の描写により、読者は著者自身のことやうつ病が著者の人生にどのような影響をおよぼしたかをより深く知ることができる。うつ病についてのこの簡潔で控えめな描写は、うつ病のまとっている未知のベールを取り払い、愛する人々がうつ病になったとしたら、あるいは今まさにうつ病で悩んでいるとしたら、その人たちにどのようなことが起こるのかを読者に伝える手がかりになるものと確信する。

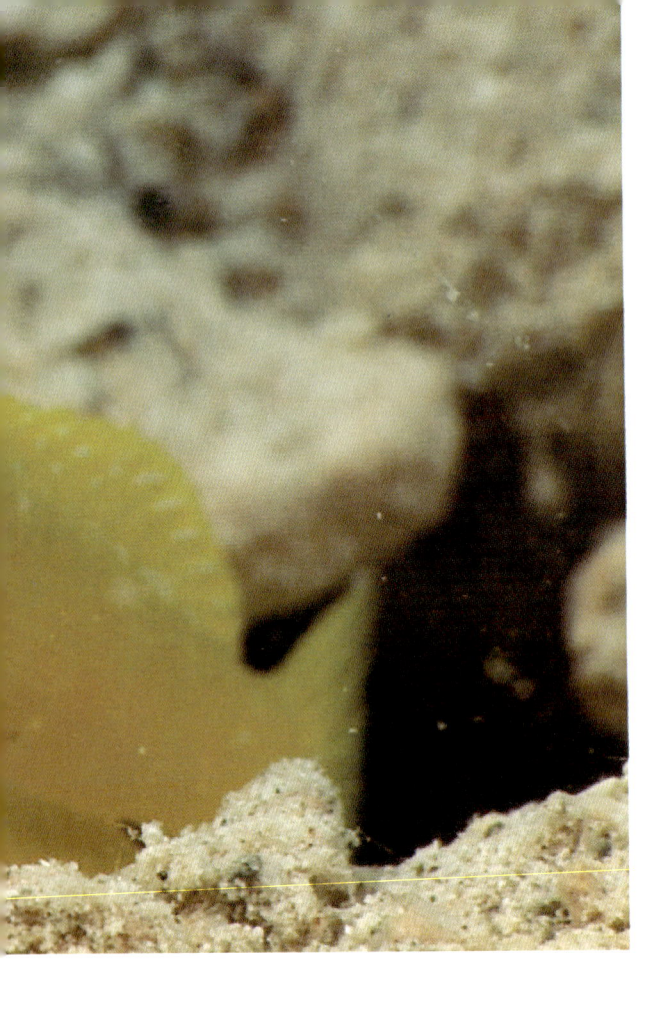

p.86 Blue Holes - Dark Space
p.88 Juvenile Batfish - A New Beginning
p.89 Brenny - Small
p.90 Underwater Cameraman, Mark Thorpe (Mr. T)
p.91 Manta Ray - Grace and Fluidity
p.91 Turtle - Defiance and Strength
p.92 Barracudas in Blue - Being Hunted
p.93 Yellow Goby - Independence
p.93 Big Drop Shallows - One the Edge
p.94 Baitball - Hunters Surrounding
p.96 Anemones Fish - Close Study
p.97 Toby - Watching for Change
p.98 Gold Goby - Starting to Shine

The images are video taken from a Sony HVR-Z1U 3CCD HDV Camcorder.

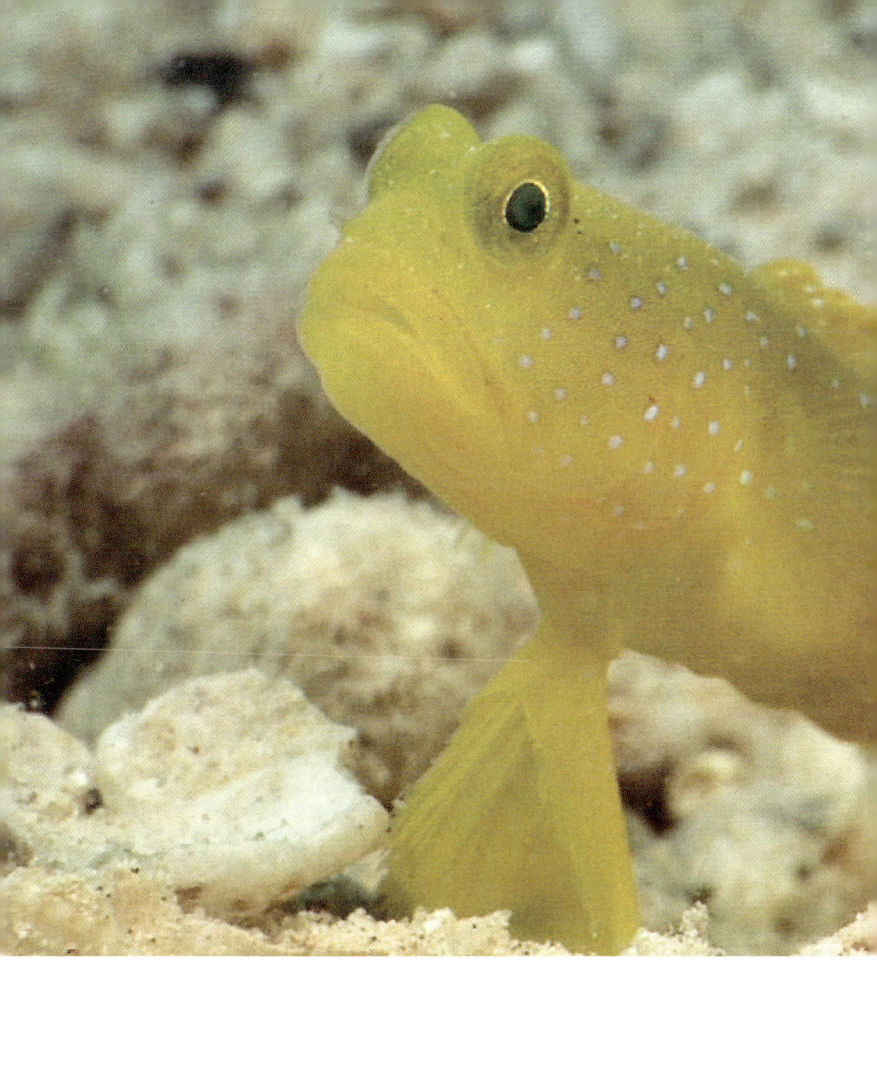

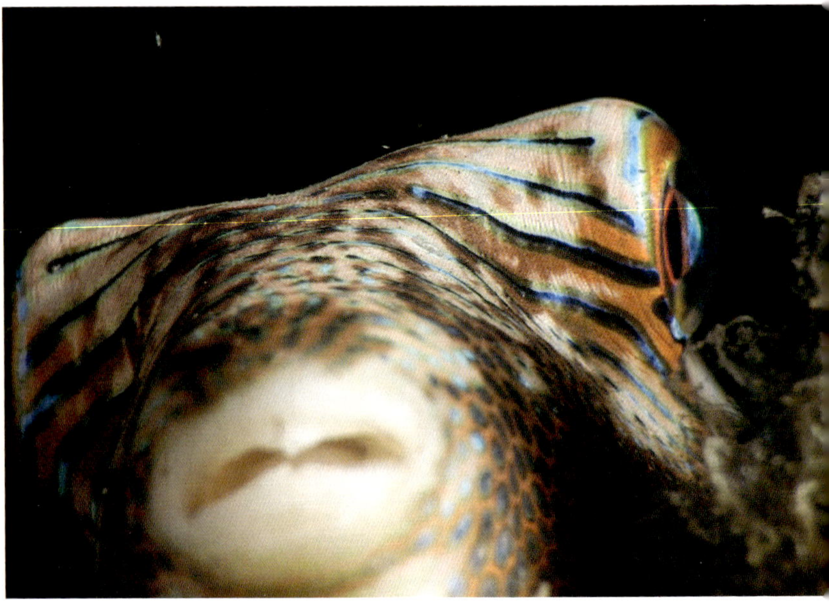

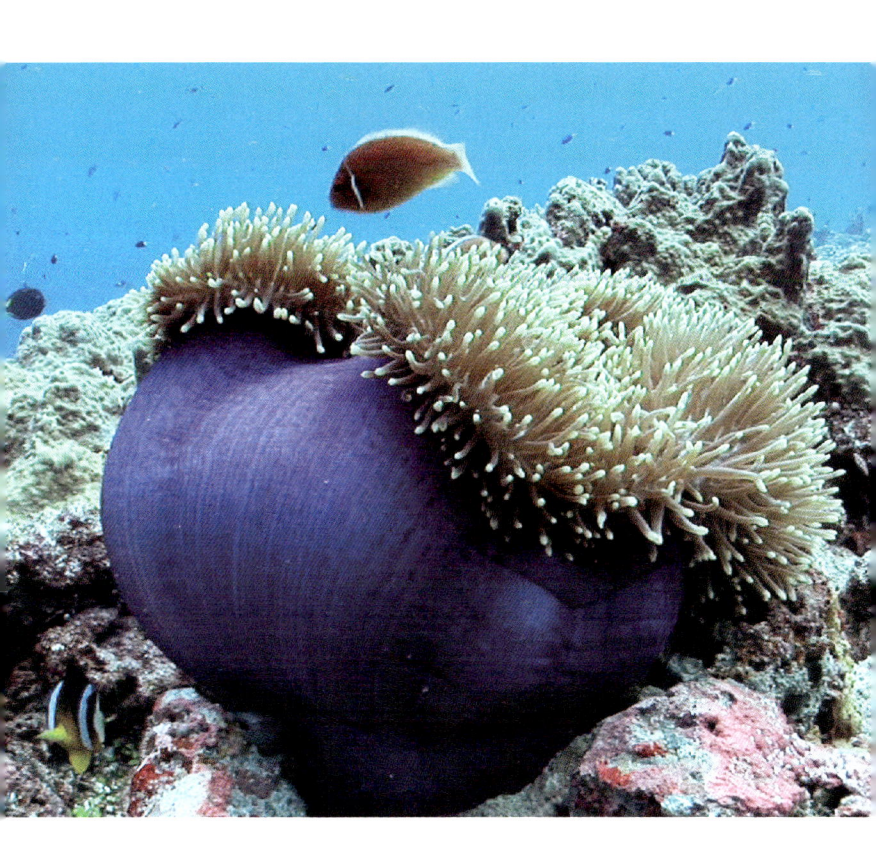

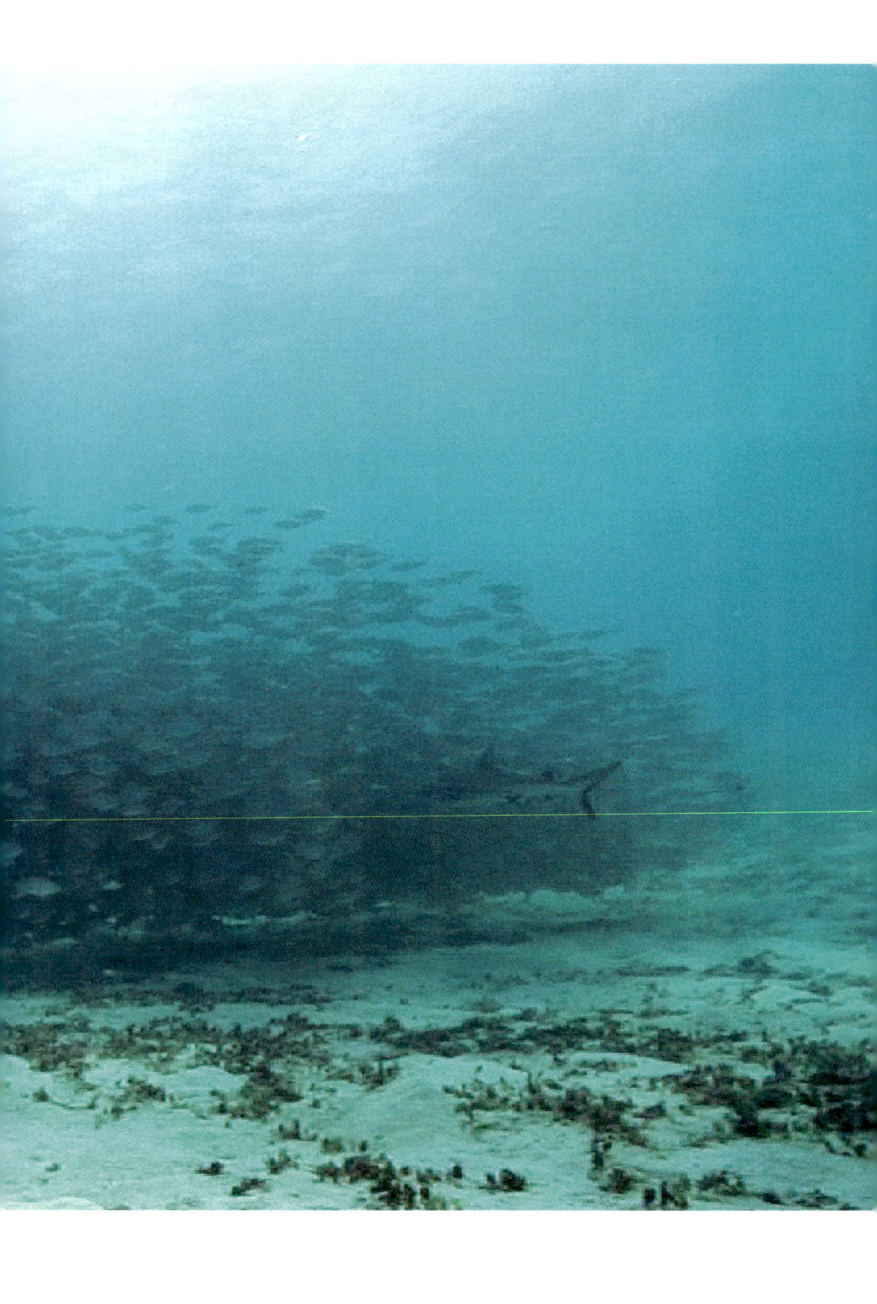

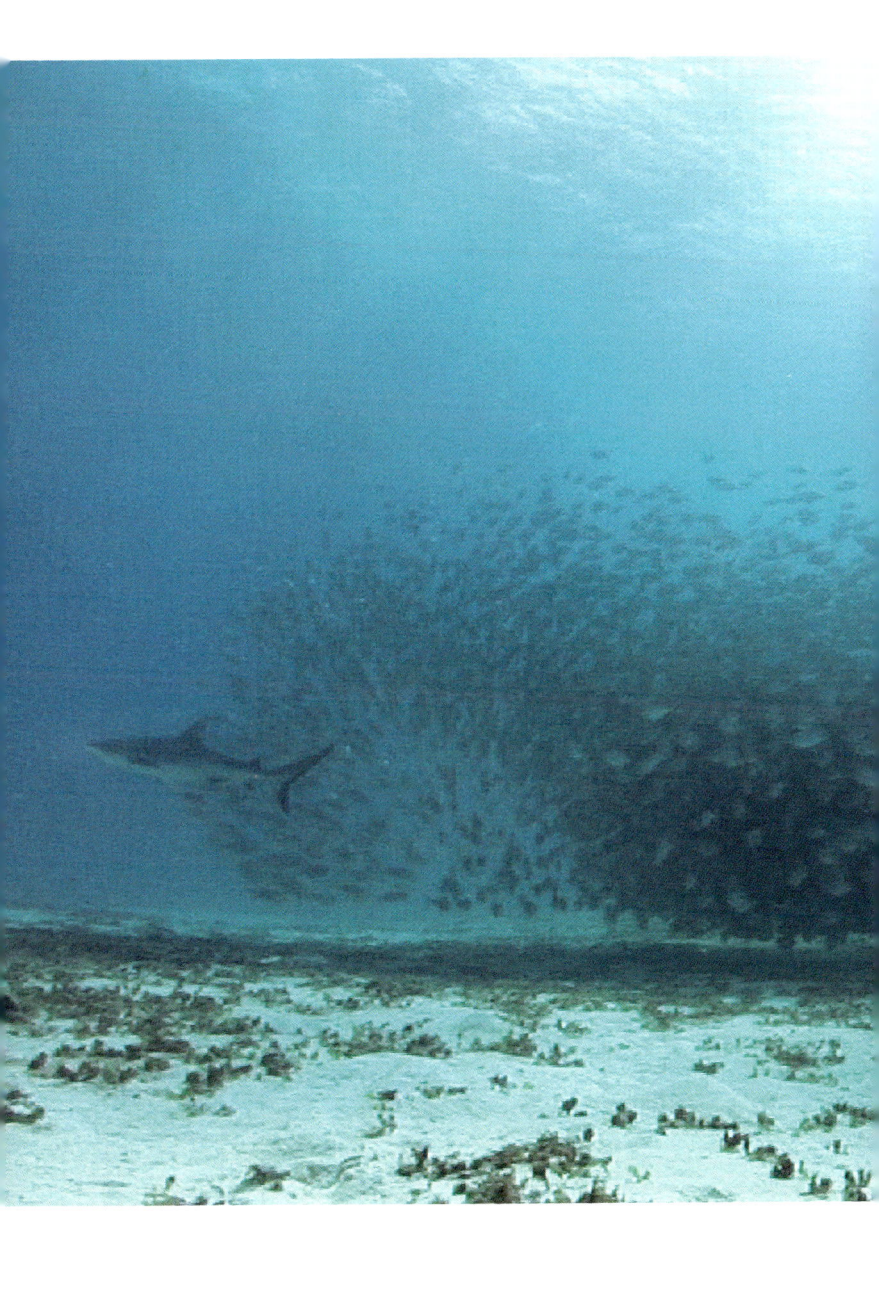

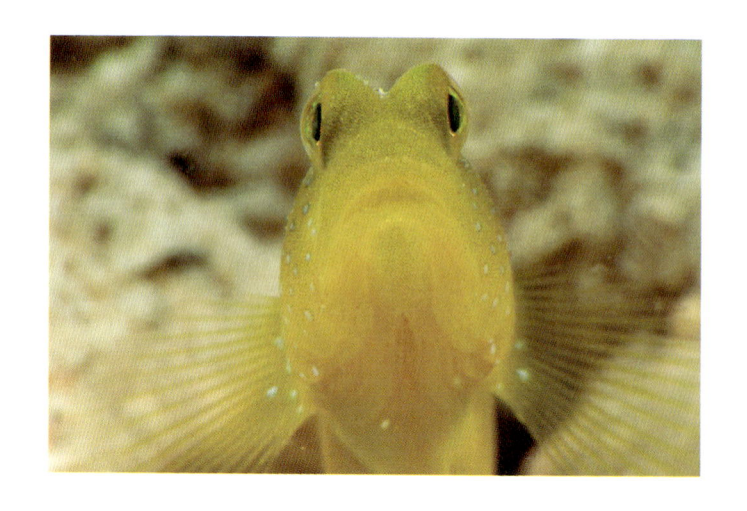

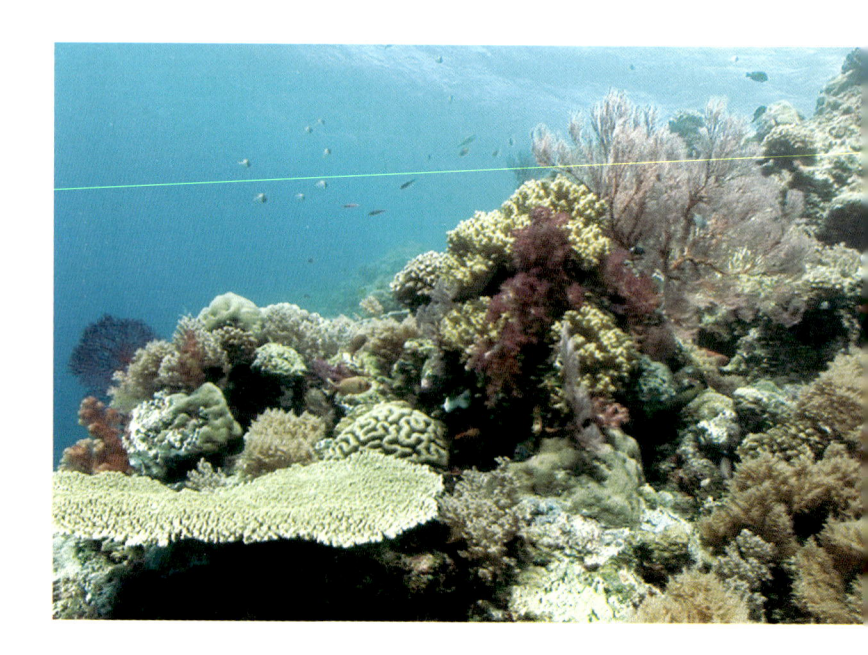

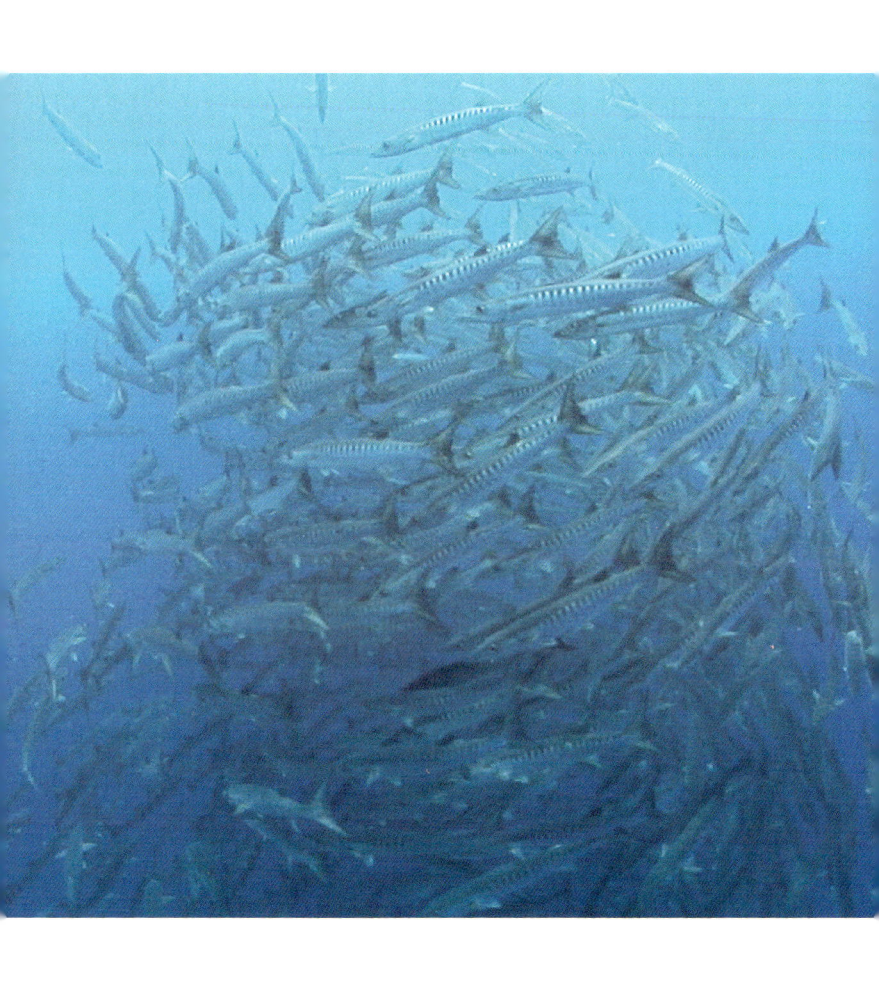

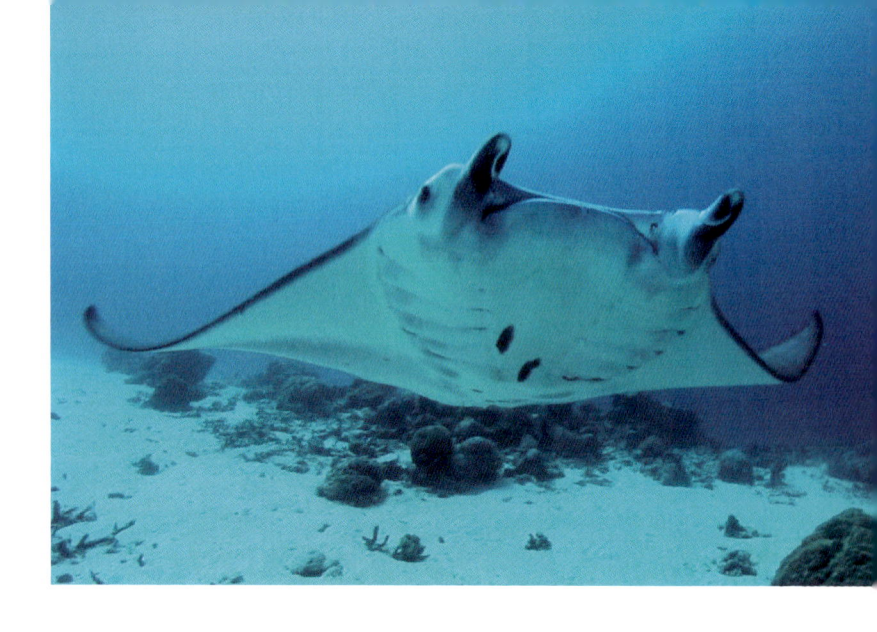

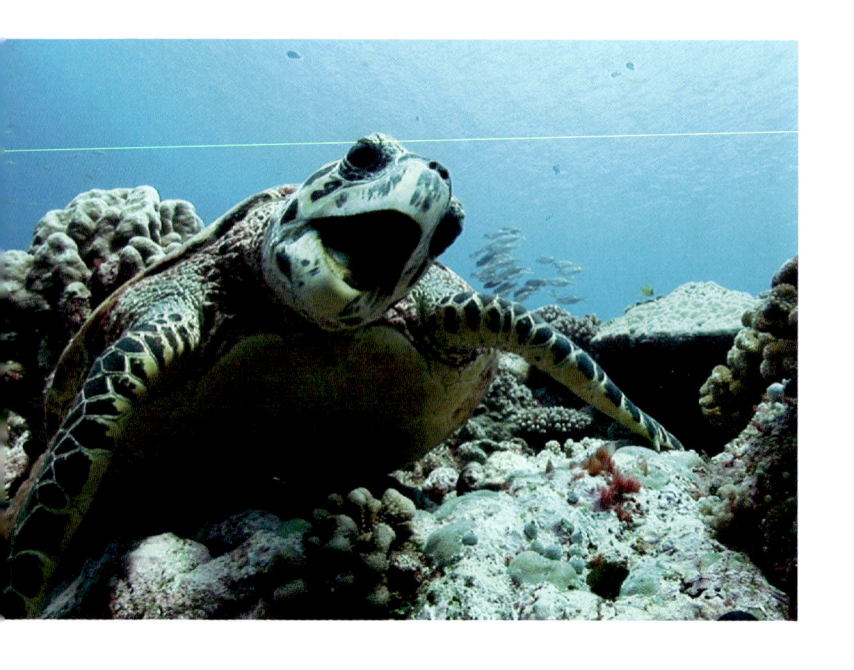

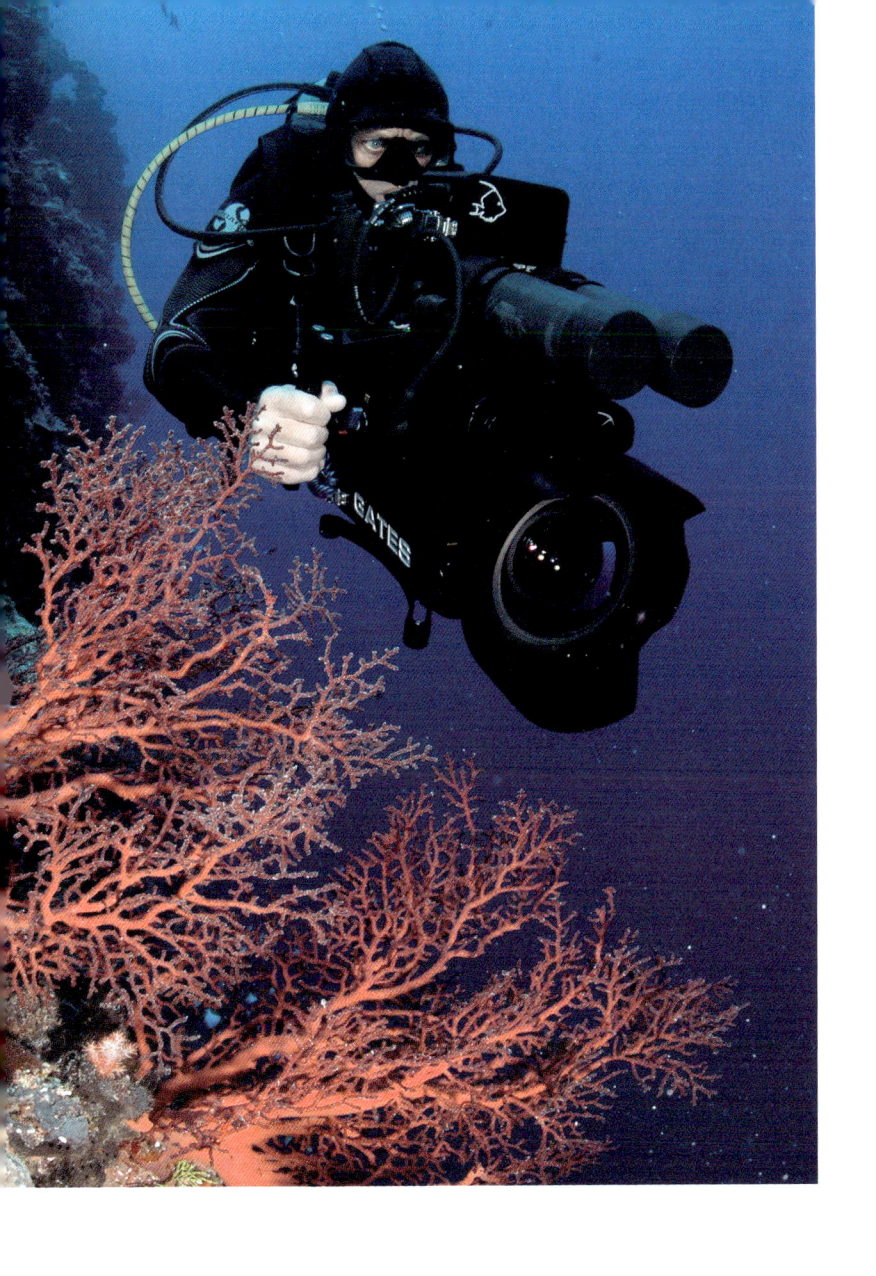

89

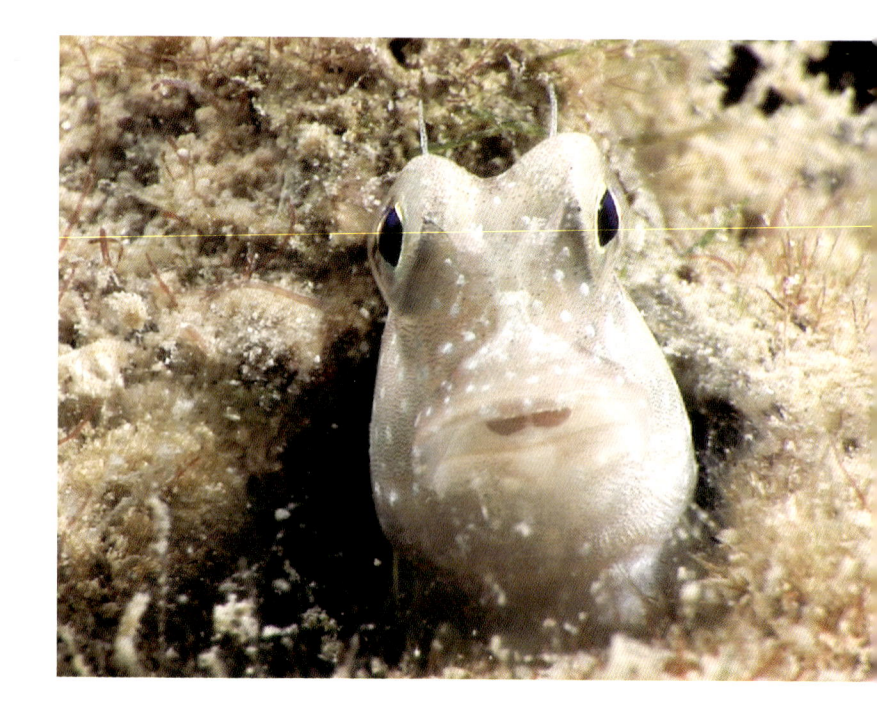

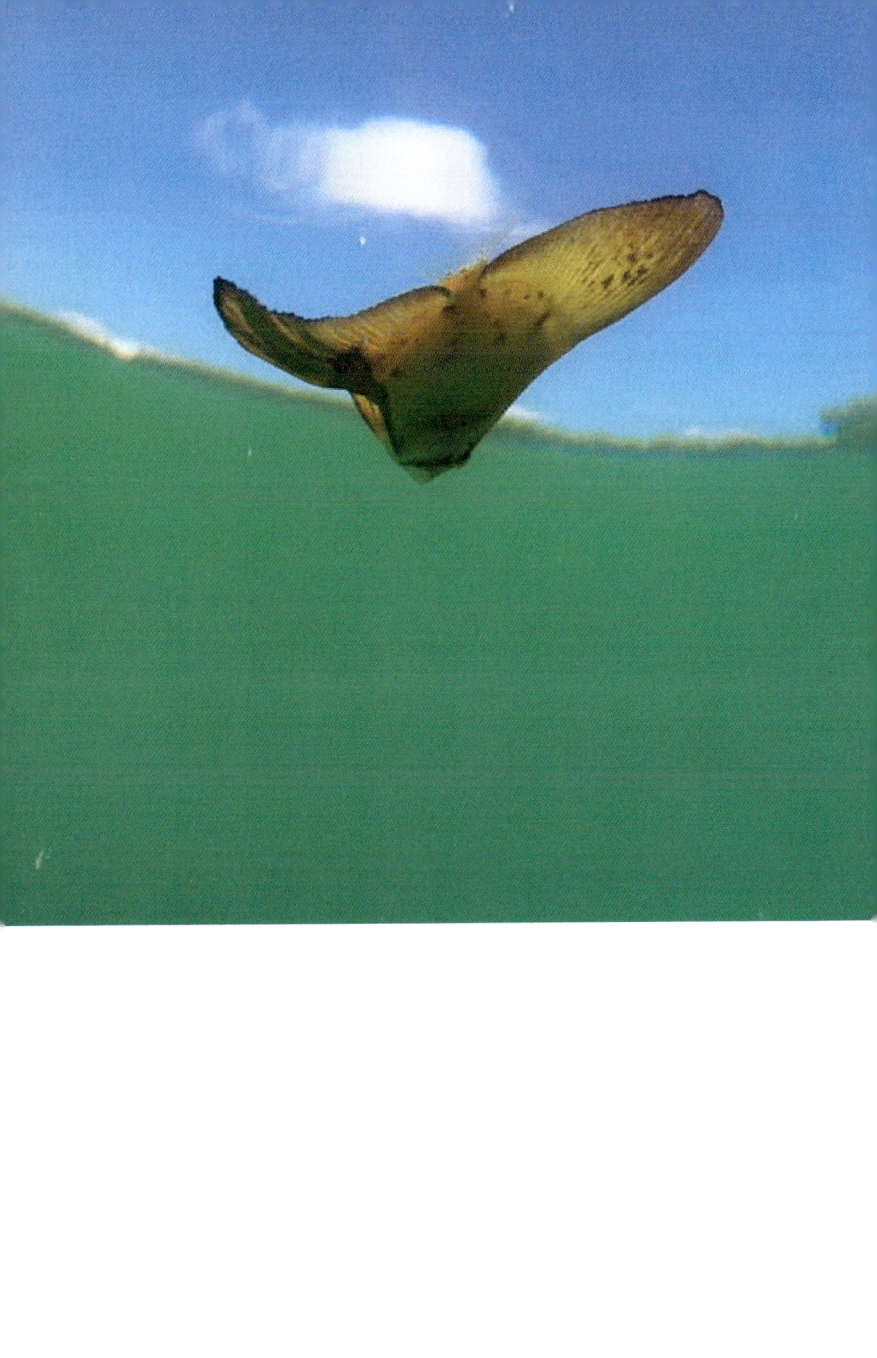

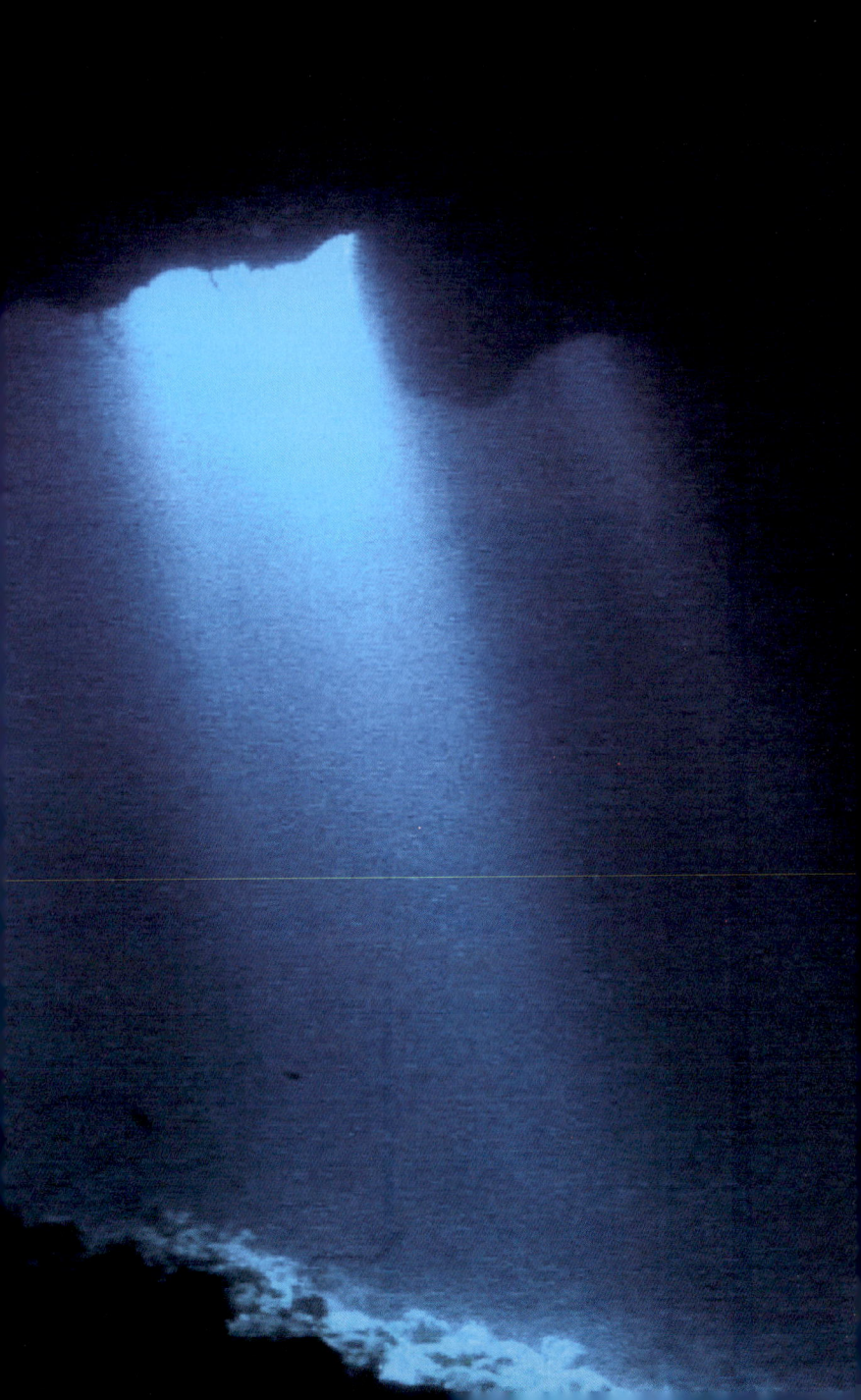

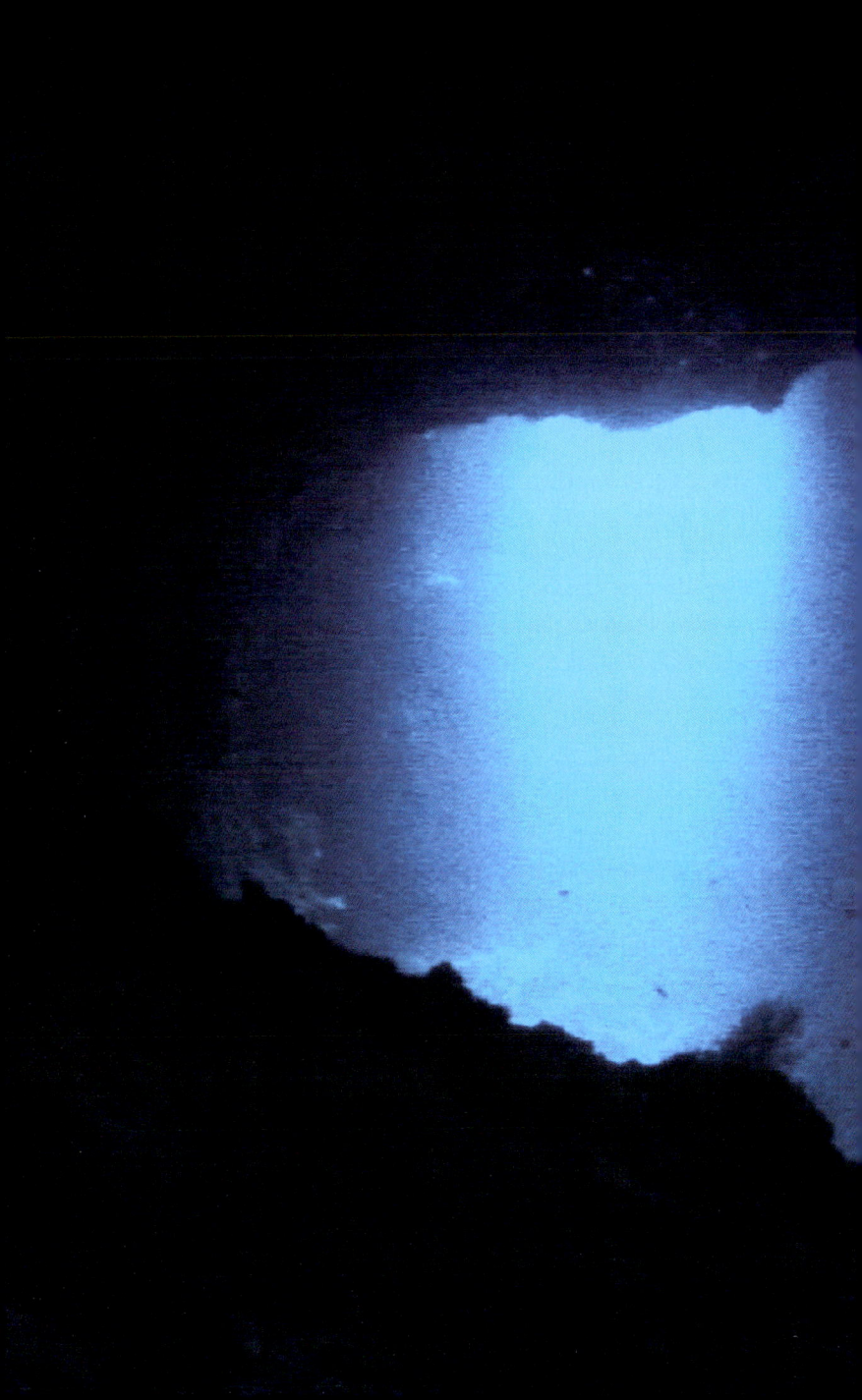

About the translator
Lee Dancy

Lee Dancy became interested in Japan while a student at the University of California at Berkeley. He started working full-time as a translator shortly after first coming to Japan in 1988. He currently lives in Hokkaido, Japan with his wife and 3 children.

Message from the translator

Prior to translating "*an ordinary psychiatrist? – navigating the darkness of depression –*" I had never even read a first-hand account of depression. Reading this story, what struck me the most was the simplicity with which it is told: I felt as if I were hearing a friend I had known all my life describe something that had happened to her. The inclusion of personal details, such as the author's love of diving and books, that at first glance would not seem to be relevant to a discussion of depression, instead serves a valuable purpose in that it prevents the disease, rather than the author as a human being, from becoming the focus of the narrative. The presentation of the author as someone with a life that is not defined solely by her depression allows the reader to acquire a more complete understanding both of the author herself and of how her life was affected by her depression. I believe that this simple, humble depiction of depression goes some way towards demystifying it and lets the reader see how it might affect, or might even now be affecting, someone they love.

continue to immerse herself in Palau's natural beauty to aid her in her recovery, so that she may eventually be reborn, as alive and vital as before, like a phoenix from the ashes.

and now spent his time on an island in the South Seas, working as a marine biologist, surrounded by nature and chasing his dreams. I, of course, am that old soldier. I gave her my opinion: "Depression is a disease of civilization: one in three people have it, they just don't realize it."

I have never liked doctors, so I don't like going to the hospital. However, I have reached the age where I am going to have to start relying on them, whether I like it or not. Yet, ironically, this psychiatrist had relied on me for help. But how much had I really been able to help her? In her story, she praises me almost as some sort of savior, but nothing could be further from the truth.

I think psychiatry must be the most difficult field of medicine. A psychiatrist has to discern the unseen contours of someone's inner thoughts and make an accurate diagnosis based solely on speech and behavior that could be considered either normal or abnormal, depending on the context. It is completely different from the kind of medicine in which someone can be treated by, for example, cutting away diseased tissue that is visible to the naked eye.

It has been several months since I first met the author and now, every time we meet, I can see that she continues to get better and better. I do hope, however, that she will cries of Tiger Finches, Giant White-eyes, Rusty-winged Starlings, and White-collared Kingfishers. However, the ring of that same telephone now echoes through the silence, and when I pick up the receiver I hear the distinctive beep indicating an incoming international call. I feel a moment of anticipation as I wait to be connected to the outside, the world beyond Palau, and then I hear a voice belonging to someone three thousand kilometers away, in Japan.

Several months earlier, the owner of that same voice, a psychiatrist by training, had visited me at my office on Palau in search of information. We talked about whales and dugongs, and I told her stories about what Palau had been like in primitive times, and also stories from my past, about larger-than-life professors from my youthful days at the Tropical Biology Institute. The second time she came to Palau, she handed me a draft of a book she said she had written, and asked me to read it. Looking at the cover, I saw that the title was "An Ordinary Psychiatrist? – Navigating the Darkness of Depression." Skimming through it, I saw that it talked about the depression that she herself had been suffering, including detailed descriptions of her symptoms, the course of her depression and, finally, her process of recovery. Towards the end, there was a passage that caught my eye. It told of her meeting a young soldier (now an old man) who had survived a great war on a deserted island. The old soldier had left Japan behind,

The Lost Phoenix —————————— Yoji Kurata

I awake to an early-morning squall. Stepping out onto the veranda, I am greeted by the dawn sky. It is five-twenty in the morning. The sky in the east is suffused with a pale light. The cattle egrets are just leaving their nests for their feeding grounds. Sometimes I only see one or two, sometimes forty or fifty at once; in a span of about thirty minutes, I can normally count about one hundred and fifty. Since we entered March two days ago, however, I have not seen a single one. They have probably left for Japan: three thousand kilometers, under their own power, and they don't even need a passport. I am envious. (A young Japanese soldier who ended up starving to death here on Palau from malnutrition wrote in the diary he left behind that "I want to return to Japan so badly I would even walk home – if only I could walk on water.")

At eight, I look to the south. I see the green, jagged mountains, the blue sea, and a lone, White-Tailed Tropicbird gliding through the sky, trailing a long, slender white tail behind it: these are the familiar sights that greet me as I begin my daily bird-watching ritual. I even lower the ring volume on my telephone so that I can catch the and despair I can only hope through our discussions there now exists hope and promise. I will continue to be available as a supporting friend and confidant.

graph of my "Happy Path" showing the high and low points of my life, which fortunately revealed more highs than lows. I believe the human mind is selective in its re-collective qualities. I mean, if I think back to, let's say, my childhood, I remember good things, episodes that bring a smile to my face. It's with a small amount of effort that I can start to recollect the bad side of those same situations. The "Happy Path" I guess is the name attributed to that initial recollection of memories.

My highs are easily obtainable, as the simple things in life leave bigger impressions on me. I am more than happy with my own company, I don't yearn for all the trappings of modern life, I am not a collector of comfort items. My life is simple, the best way for me.

I can only base my personal take on life by the experiences I have been fortunate or unfortunate, as the case may be, to have witnessed first hand. I believe we all, as a race, have the ability to rationalize, to love and to appreciate the true spirit of humanity. It just takes a bit more effort from some as opposed to others but it is there and ready to be discovered in all of us. I have found my happiness beneath the waves, and I will continue to do what I love so long as I feel that this is what drives me.

My friendship with the author is a continued one of deep trust and appreciation. Where there was once doubt de la Legion Etrangere) for two years and it was here that I found my calling.

Learning to dive on a whim after a brief chat with one of the French guys in my section I found a world beneath the Red Sea where I felt free. It was like nothing else I had ever experienced in my life. I had always been fascinated with nature as a child. We lived close to a forest in the south of England so I would always find myself jumping across brooks and searching for Newts or snakes on the common ground. Diving through the pristine reefs of Djibouti gave me reason, gave me freedom but above all it gave me hope. I wished the final years of my military service away and then embarked on the career in which I now find myself.

Having read this story of confinement and darkness I could relate to the feelings of depression as my friend poured her heart out. I never considered my experience in life to be a depressive one but I guess it all depends on how the individual perceives depression. Some have stronger thresholds than others. I guess I never had a benchmark to set against so I wouldn't have even known if I was depressed or not, I don't think I was. One thing I was very aware of though was the massive weight that seemed to be lifted from me once I started out on my non-military calling. I could see the darkness of certain past events in my life and used them to draw an imaginary

This was the start of my slow transition into seeking peace and quiet in an environment devoid of the violence and hatred we see perpetrated on a daily basis around our slowly spinning planet. How could there be so much hatred, so much hatred to warrant the blowing up, the ritual assassinations, the decapitations of our fellow man. How could some people warrant metering out that kind of pain on each other was beyond me. Yet here I was in the middle of it all. This was bedlam. I witnessed riots, bombings, murders and fanaticism on many levels.

The years in the military seemed to gel into one continued period of numbness. I awoke one day to find that I had even changed allegiance to the hand that fed me. Speaking French and wearing the flaming grenade cap badge of the French Foreign Legion I had left the British Infantry and was now serving in this mystical outfit of nationals and expatriates, each with our differing reasons and convictions. It was deemed as 'incorrect' to ask fellow Legionnaires the reasons for their serving with the various units of the Legion so I just went along with it and basked in my own anonymity. There were a few ex-British military guys that I got along with but we mainly just co-existed with each other purely for no other reason than the ability to be able to communicate with one another outside of regular "Office Hours". I served in Djibouti in the horn of Africa as my first posting. I had been effected to the 13eme D.B.L.E (13eme Demi Brigade grandmother or with foster parents. Neither of these options seemed to work for us so for me, from the age of six, my "family" was comprised of many tens of other kids in similar situations as my sister and I. Needless to say the relationship that developed between my sister and I was a far cry from the close relationship one would have cultivated in a normal family environment. There was just too much going on. We understood and recognized each other but we just didn't have the chance to develop a close relationship. With no other brothers and sisters I started to consider myself, from a very early age, as being alone and answerable only to myself.

Joining the military at age 16 was a choice almost made for me by the social services policy at the time in the U.K. I had been told that if by the time I was 17 I had no job then I would basically be forced to leave this custodial environment and forge a life on my own. Needless to say I signed military papers once I had achieved sufficient grades in the aptitude exams. So here I was entering, albeit this time voluntarily, into another 'institution'. A protective environment, there were not that many wars to fight as there are today, cocooning me from the reality of modern day responsibilities. I was safe here, or at least that's what I thought.

Walking the streets of Belfast as an 18 year old Infantry soldier in the early 1980's was an eye opening experience.

| **Reflections** ──────────── Mark Thorpe |

The four pilot whales split away from the main herd and came straight at me. The air pocket in my chest cavity reverberated with their sonar as they approached. Their inquisitiveness at this strange being in their midst had gotten the better of them and they were here to investigate. Passing just feet away from me all I could do was marvel at their agility and speed, they had closed a gap of ten meters that had existed between themselves and I within seconds. I also knew that these were intelligent animals, I could see that as I stared deep into their inky black eyes. I was also very much aware that if they wished they had the power, both individually and collectively, to end my very existence right there, right then. But they chose not to. Instead I found myself sharing one of those what I term as "Magic Moments" with an intelligent being in an environment alien to that to which I was accustomed. The aquatic environment, to me, feels more like home than the one we as a species call our own.

I had grown up in nationally subsidised child-care facilities on the south coast of England. Both my sister and I had started our respective lives either in the care of our

new day will surely dawn. If you can get yourself to walk down the street and turn the corner, you will be greeted by a scene, a vision, you haven't seen before. Each day is different from the next. Although your physical existence might remain unchanged, you live a new reality each and every day.

Looking back on my experience, I can safely say that I don't ever want to become depressed again. I lost something that I will never get back. Moreover, I know that, with depression, it is all too easy to have a relapse. No one can say for sure if they will experience depression only once in their life, or several times. However, I know that, even if I become depressed once again, the experience and knowledge that I have gained by having lived through it once will prove invaluable for getting me through it the next time.

Furthermore, by experiencing such suffering, I gained something, as well, for my bout with depression brought me into contact with some wonderful people and taught me things I didn't know about the warmth of the human heart. I learned about different ways of living and thinking. Perhaps I should even be thankful.

Those were peaceful mornings.

I once again became able to enjoy diving. I stopped just staring blankly into the deep blue water. When I went diving with Mr. T, I was able to enjoy my own dive experience without being a burden to him. I felt as if, when Mr. T and I were underwater, we instinctively knew what each other was thinking, without having to verbalize our thoughts or even communicate them nonverbally in any way – we were just naturally on the same wavelength. For me, this was wonderful beyond words.

Illustrations of fish, turtles, manta rays, and other sea creatures once again began appearing in my log book. I started coloring in my illustrations again, and looking up the names of each species in an illustrated field guide and writing them down in my logs.

The scenes that left the biggest impression on me were those of animals that clung to life despite being injured: a turtle with a mangled right hind leg; an eagle ray with a deformed, bent tail; a manta ray with a tail torn off at the base. Had they been attacked by predators, and yet still managed to escape and live on? I even saw the eagle ray with the deformed tail a second time, at a different dive site.

At any rate, the important thing, for them as well as us, is to keep on living. If you can just manage to hold on, a

20

Epilogue

One day, I came across a pamphlet for an antidepressant medication that resonated with me, and I had it pinned up over my desk for a while. It showed a picture of a woman standing in front of a sink in the morning wearing a white bathrobe and brushing her teeth. A light brown tabby cat was perched on top of the sink, looking up at the woman's face with a satisfied grin that brought to mind my own cat's purring. The text said something like "A Cheerful Mood for a Pleasant Morning." At the time, I didn't really know why I liked that image so much, but now, after having experienced depression, I know that it captures with uncanny accuracy the way one feels when one's "morning depression" has lifted.

I, too, have recovered my ability to greet the morning with a smile, at least most of the time. By coincidence, just like tha cat in the pamphlet, my cat would also jump up onto the sink while I was brushing my teeth, and rub her forehead against by body. It seemed that my cat thought that the proper way to greet me in the morning was to press her forehead against mine, and she would pace back and forth on top of the sink trying to get my attention, waiting for me to crouch down to greet her.

sorts, even in this state, there were people who were willing to accept me as a friend. Those people let me know they were worried about me without being pushy. They would call me, and be with me only for as long as I could handle it. Just knowing that those people were worrying about me was helpful because, when I was going through a tough spell, I would remember that there were people who cared about me, even as I was. Just knowing that was comforting.

It may take some time before you find people you can count on for support. In fact, it doesn't even have to be a person – animals make wonderful companions that can bring you great comfort in times of need. When I was unable to get out of bed for practically the entire day, my cat would lie by my side for hours on end, keeping me company (not necessarily because it was being nice, of course – maybe just out of habit, but still …). When I would reach out and stroke her soft, fluffy, warm fur, she would purr quietly. On those nights when I couldn't get to sleep, I would listen to the sound of her quiet breathing, and sometimes she would even talk in her sleep.

Also, if you can find pictures, books, or music that can ease the pain of your depression, then they can become your companions. They will speak to you, if you are willing to listen to what they have to say.

lean on for support. Of course, when they start treatment, their doctors will support them. However, since their doctors are not going to be available all the time, patients need to find as many different people as possible on whom they can rely for support. People who become depressed may receive support from people from whom they least expect it. People who the patient did not think would be so kind or concerned often step up to help out. For this reason, it is important to keep one's heart open at all times, to accept help no matter who it is from.

By the same token, people that the patient had expected to be there for support or that had been close up until then sometimes become cold, indifferent, and aloof, always keeping their distance; I experienced this myself. Sometimes I would explain what I was going through over and over and still some people would not understand. And then there were people who tried to push their kindness on me because of some self-centered, ulterior motive. I was already more sensitive to, and even fearful of, my relationships with other people because of my depression, and such unpleasant encounters made me feel even worse. It was precisely at such times when I would find out exactly who was really concerned about me.

Even though I had become unable to work, even though I was glum and negative, even though I would always mope about things and had no energy, even though I was irritable and cranky, even though I was mentally out of

I could finally see the light at the end of the tunnel.

19

Someone to Lean On

I mentioned before that once someone's depression exceeds a certain level of severity, that person must get rest and must start taking an antidepressant medication, and that having people to lean on for support is equally important. Normally, the first candidates that come to mind are family members. I think patients with family members who are kind to and protective of them are very lucky.

However, not everyone is so lucky. Some patients do not have any family members who will stand by them, and many patients live alone. Unfortunately, there are also times when a patient's family will not be able to understand depression or will hold a prejudiced opinion of it. There are also people who either do not want to believe, or else cannot accept, that someone from their own family is clinically depressed.

Even if patients have no close family members, or no one in their family can understand what they are going through, they will always be able to find someone they can hospital and, for patients I am seeing for the first time, to help lighten the anxiety, anger, and distress they naturally feel on their first visit, is to try to get each patient to laugh before the visit is over. It is possible to make someone laugh without telling jokes or being witty. I often make myself the butt of the jokes. Moreover, even if I am not able to make them laugh, I resolve to try to not let any crying or angry patients go home without first getting them in a better mood.

In the field of psychiatry, quite a few patients cry in the doctor's office. Boxes of tissue are placed in each consultation room, and they are not there for people with colds. They are there so that they can be reached at a moment's notice when a patient starts to cry. Those tissue boxes get used a lot.

If someone can laugh from the bottom of their heart, in that moment, their heart will feel lighter, as if it had been cleansed somehow. The healing power of laughter is discussed in "How to Laugh Like a Professional," as well. Laughter accompanied by joyful, happy, pleasant emotions is extremely important to everyone, and can serve as a barometer for the severity of one's depression. Seeing myself laughing from the heart made me breathe a little easier about my own depression. Once I was able to laugh like that not just once, but on several different occasions, I felt as if everything around me had just gotten a little brighter.

looking for. Thanks to my improving condition, I was finally able to do this kind of "bookstore hopping" again.

It was in this way that I became able to really laugh again. I then remembered, a little late, something that I had always made sure to do when I was treating patients, which was to always make them laugh, if possible, before letting them out of my office. In the field of psychiatry, there are many patients who need to be treated on an outpatient basis for a long time. When I would review their voluminous medical histories, spanning several, or even 10 or more, years, divided up into separate binders when one was not enough, it would make me think about how much stress they must have been feeling all along to have to come to the hospital and take medication for so many years. I do not ask patients I have been treating for a long time about their symptoms, particularly if it is not necessary. Patients who really want to talk about their symptoms will, even if doing so means interrupting my attempts at small talk. Some patients endure in silence without talking about their symptoms, even if they are feeling very poorly, some patients tell me about their symptoms in detail, and some pay too much attention to their symptoms; as a doctor, you get a feel for each patient's individual personality over the years.

Therefore, what I do for patients I have been treating for a long time to help relieve the stress of coming to the professional speaking down to amateurs, but was instead treating his audience as his equals, giving them detailed insight into the world of traditional Japanese performance art. And the lecture itself was extremely interesting. Although I am ashamed to admit it, my only previous exposure to *Rakugo* had been on one or two occasions when I was a child, and I didn't remember the names of the performers or what stories they had told. Yet even I, who had no real appreciation for the art, became totally engrossed, and I couldn't put the book down.

And then, I started laughing, without even trying to. I felt like I would be able to read the whole book at one sitting, but I caught myself and, remembering how tired I would be the next day if I went ahead and read the whole book, I put it aside, albeit a little reluctantly.

I knew that I would regret it if I read the book through to the end. The next day, I went out to take care of a few things so, while I was out, I stopped by a few bookstores and bought all of the books written by that author that I could find. Only then did I finish reading the first book.

Of course, nowadays you can order any book you want over the internet. With just one click, you can even have it express mailed to you the next day. However, going to a bookstore in person is an entirely different experience than ordering books over the internet and, for a bookworm like me, there is no greater joy than making the rounds of the different bookstores and finally finding the books I'm be able to do anything more than buy diving magazines with lots of pictures, so I had stopped going. I don't know why, but that day, I suddenly felt like looking for some interesting books.

I went to *Yakumodo*, a small, cozy bookstore. Standing there, looking at the rows of books that had once been such a familiar sight, I felt a little nostalgic. If I had gone to the bookstore earlier, when I wasn't able to concentrate on things, I would have been able to focus enough to read the titles of all the books lined up on the shelves. That day, however, I was able to stay focused and search for interesting books. One book caught my eye. It was a compilation of lectures that had been given at Keio University by Katsura Bunchin, a famous *Rakugo* (traditional Japanese comic storytelling) performance artist, entitled "How to Laugh Like a Professional." Normally, I would buy several books, but that day I bought just that one, and then went back home.

When I opened the book and started reading, I realized that the author was indeed a master storyteller: I immediately felt as if I had been transported to the lecture hall in which he had originally given the speeches, and was sitting alongside all of the hundreds of students who had gone to see him speak. His ability to set the scene, to get the audience interested and involved, and to establish the proper pacing for his stories, was magical. Moreover, he did not seem to be putting himself on a pedestal , as a as always, that nothing is wrong, so much so that there is even a term for this: "smiling depression."

However, when people who are depressed become unable to keep up appearances in this way, they no longer want to be around anyone else. Then, if their depression gets even worse, they become terrified of crowds or of simply passing strangers on the street. It gets to the point where they can't leave home.

The English word "personality" derives from the Greek word "persona," which means "mask." You, and everyone else, without exception, put on a mask – the "you that you present to others" – when you are with other people. Putting on this mask is hard work if you are depressed. And yet, without this mask, you feel extremely fragile and defenseless, as if you will be damaged beyond repair if you are hurt by others while in this state, and this is why you can no longer be around other people.

For the longest time, I was not able to laugh or have a good time; indeed, I felt as if laughing or having a good time was almost inconceivable. However, shortly after I started having "normal mornings" again, one day I suddenly had the urge to go to a bookstore. I had always liked books and, before I had become depressed, I had been in the habit of going to a bookstore about 3 times a week. At that point, however, I hadn't been even once in I don't know how many weeks. I had known that I wouldn't optimistically: for example, by being willing to just lie down and get a little rest to take the edge off of the fatigue, rather than trying to fight through it.

18

Laughter

When someone is depressed, they can't enjoy anything. You could say that a person has become severely depressed if they can no longer enjoy the things they used to like the most. Before people reach that point, they often go through a period where they can still enjoy doing things they like, but they can no longer work effectively. It is not that these people are being lazy – it is simply a matter of the degree of severity of the depression. However, when someone can no longer enjoy something he or she normally greatly enjoys, that is a sign that the depression has reached all the way down to the bottom of their heart.

If the person is able to go out and meet people – in other words, unless the person is confined to bed at home – they might be able to put on a happy face when they are around others. However, that is only because they are trying hard to hide their condition, not because they are really happy or having fun. Depressed people are often trying to put on a brave face, trying to show others that they are the same was starting to roll forward. I was also aware that I was now thinking more quickly (although admittedly not as quick as before). I was also getting better at complex, intricate tasks. Moreover, once I had decided to do something, I no longer worried too much about whether or not it was a mistake.

I could tell, when I looked in the mirror, that my expression had become more relayed and confident. My tone of voice and the pace of my conversation were also changing. When I was having a bad day, I would appear either lifeless and apathetic – like a shadow of myself – or else irritable and angry. My voice would become quiet, and my speech would slow.

When you are involved with the same patients for many years, you can tell the moment you open the door and they step into your office whether they are having a good or a bad day. I had started to change enough that, when I was having a bad day, other people could tell the difference, too.

Of course, that did not mean that I was having good days all the time. There were days when I felt bad, and could not concentrate, from the moment I got up. There were also times when I was abnormally sleepy and listless. However, I had reached the point where that did not bother me; I accepted that this was just the way it was going to be. Since I truly believed that I was really headed in the right direction, I was able to deal with such setbacks originally been an avid walker who had become unable to go walking because of his depression, and he said that, since he had started feeling better, he had gone walking in order to try to finally start getting some exercise again. I was surprised. Even when healthy, I am not the type of person who can go walking for 4 hours. And he had been staying at home in bed for a long time up until just a few weeks before.

I told him that of course he was going to get tired and have to retreat to bed if he went walking for 4 hours a day, that that didn't mean that his depression had gotten worse, and that I didn't mind if he started walking again, but that he should at least keep it down to 1 hour, and stop before he got tired. While this is an extreme example, it is very common for patients to suddenly let down their guard and try to do too much when they are just starting to get better. In order to recover from depression without suffering major setbacks like this, you need to have the courage to stop yourself from doing things just because you have suddenly recovered the ability to do them.

I had reached the point where, after I got up in the morning and had thought about my schedule for the day, I could actually do some work, or read a book. The sluggishness of my thoughts – "thought inhibition," in medical terms – had begun to lift and, like a car that had been parked, the ignition to the engine of my mind had been turned on, the parking brake had been released, and I everything I was thinking about doing that day, it would be too much for me to handle, so I would know to put it off until the following day. I had become much better able to prioritize, although still not as well as before. When I got tired, it would take me several days to recover, so I needed to stop myself. I resolved to do no more than one thing a day.

I was always telling my patients "only do half as much as you think you can," but I was starting to realize just how hard it was to follow my own advice. Until you get better, you can't think about what you are going to do in an orderly fashion, nor can you really figure out how to pace yourself so that your workload is in line with what you can actually do.

One of my patients had gotten much better, but then had an episode that is all too common. Until one day, he had been coming along nicely. However, at one visit, he said that he had felt good in the first half of the week, but then had become very tired, and had been staying in bed the whole second half of the week. He had originally become depressed due to intense fatigue and, with treatment, he had gradually become able to stay out of bed for longer and longer each day. Why, then, did he suddenly have such a recurrence?

When I asked him whether or not something had triggered this episode, he said that he had gone walking for 4 hours a day in the first part of the week. He had was practically a cause for celebration. I thought "what a joy it is to simply be able to wake up normally in the morning."

From that day on, I started having more and more days when I was able to just "wake up normally." That day marked when the higher dosage I was on started working. My powers of concentration gradually returned to normal, as well. I started being able to accurately judge how long it would take me to do things based on the nature of the work, as long as it was something with which I was familiar. In other words, I regained my ability to estimate time: this will take 3 days, that will take 2, that sort of thing. While I was still not back to where I had been before I became depressed, I was able to think more quickly and take care of things more easily. In addition, while I would still wonder how I was going to get through the day on my bad days, on my "normal days," I was now able to run through the day's schedule in my mind: "first I'll do this, and then that."

Now, on my bad days, I would either just sleep it off, or else I would be restless, and do things like just wandering around town aimlessly. However, day by day, I gradually became better at planning things and conducting my life in a more orderly fashion.

Furthermore, I was now able to think clearly about the order in which I had to do things before I started actually doing them. I was now able to recognize that, if I did effects of the antidepressant.

The first improvement I noticed after I started using a higher dose was in my insomnia. Up until then, while there had been times when I could get to sleep, there had also been times when I couldn't for hours on end, and I would get tired only after I had stayed up all night and gotten up the next morning. Every night, I had been constantly worrying before going to bed about whether or not I would be able to get to sleep. However, after I started using a higher dose, I was able to fall asleep more easily, until finally I was at least able to stop worrying about whether or not I would be able to sleep.

Then, after about 10 days had passed, something surprising happened. Until then, every morning when I woke up, I would be in a simply awful frame of mind, some sort of combination of intense sorrow, anxiety, irritability, and fatigue.

Then, one morning, I just woke up normally. I wasn't particularly anxious, nor particularly sad, nor particularly irritable or tired. In the moment after I opened my eyes, I thought "something's different." I myself, however, didn't realize what it was at first. More than anything, I suppose, it was that I felt awake. While I lay in bed wondering what was going on, I realized with a start that I didn't feel bad. I was able to get out of bed normally, and I didn't have to sit down in front of my closet. I was able to stand at the sink on my own two legs and wash my face. This improvement coming in waves, I felt like I was stuck in place, going up and down but in a circle, never moving forward, just like a rollercoaster. It seemed that the effectiveness of my medication had plateaued, just as I was on the verge of getting better.

Therefore, I decided to see what would happen if I increased my dosage. As I mentioned above, since I had not been able to use a higher dosage with the first medication that I had tried because of the side effects, I had started taking a different medication. However, apparently I should have been taking a higher dose. I had been reluctant to take a higher dose of the second medication because of the difficulties I had experienced with the first, but since it didn't seem as if I could expect to get better without trying something, I went ahead and started taking a higher dose. If I had to go off of this medication too because of side effects, I thought that I could always just switch to yet another; there are lots of antidepressants. Thinking that made me feel a little better.

Although I had been nervous about using a higher dose, this time, my side effects didn't get worse, and I was able to continue taking the medication. I had doubled my dosage and, while my side effects didn't get twice as bad, they didn't disappear, nor did I ever get used to them. There were times when I didn't notice them so much, but there were also times when they bothered me so much that I had to take a separate medication just to counter the side blaming myself, losing all hope, and thinking I would never get better, Mr. T. wrote me, and ended his letter with "I know you are going to be well." At the time, I myself wouldn't have said that I was going to be well, but I decided that, if he believed I would be well, then I probably would be. I decided that, when I couldn't trust my own thoughts, I would have to trust the opinions of the people who were helping me.

Trusting people had always been extremely difficult for me. However, thanks to my having become clinically depressed, I was slowly becoming able to trust people. I concluded that being depressed may therefore do me some good after all. And not just some minor benefit, either; maybe it would help me gain something very valuable, indeed.

17

One Morning

Although my symptoms had improved considerably compared to when I was at my lowest point, I was still stuck in my familiar pattern of ups and downs. As I described above, with depression, improvement comes in waves, and patients often suffer temporary setbacks on their road to recovery. Actually, this is the normal pattern of recovery. However, in my case, rather than

16

Trusting People

As soon as I got back to Japan, my condition got worse again. Even after I would take a day off, when I would get home from work the following day I would just crawl into bed and stay there. However, I no longer really paid any attention to my condition. There was nothing I could do about it; I just wasn't better yet. Maybe I couldn't work exactly the way I used to be able to, but one of these days I would get better. I also started to wonder why it had been necessary for me to work so much in the past. No one and nothing had been forcing me to do it. I had simply gotten it into my head at some point that my life wouldn't have any meaning or value if I didn't work so hard.

Even though I am still searching for the light at the end of the tunnel, even though I may no longer have any great expectations for myself, I have at least learned that there are indeed wonderful people living in this world, people like Dr. Sakurai, Dr. Yamada, Dr. Kurata, and Mr. T. Each of them has wonderful hopes and dreams. I feel privileged to have met them, because just having been allowed to steal a glance at their dreams has allowed me to feel joy again.

When I was lost in the dark maze of my depression,

at such ease with his graciousness that I didn't hesitate to just drop in on him. The third time I went to see him, I didn't even call first, I just went over. Dr. Kurata said, in a humorous tone, "Would you please wait a second. I just came out of the shower, and haven't had time to put on my makeup." He always managed to create such a lighthearted, joking atmosphere.

Dr. Kurata's field of expertise was sea turtles, so he told me about sea turtles, but he was also tremendously concerned with keeping records of the old traditions and history of Palau that were being lost. His home and office were both buried beneath reams of books and papers, a treasure trove of information.

After showing me around Koror, the capital of Palau, he took me to the naval cemetery there, and talked about the history of the tombstones and monuments. He pointed out that the cemetery faced north – in the direction of Japan. The view of the ocean from the sloping hill on which the cemetery stood was unforgetable. The colors seemed to be slightly faded, with everything bathed in white.

as if he were some wise old man living alone on a mountain. In addition to being extremely intelligent, he was also extremely nice. I don't know if it was because he had that preternatural tranquility that was unique to people who have lived through tragedies, but he possessed a calm strength and tremendous kindness. In that way, I felt that Mr. T. and Dr. Kurata were alike.

Dr. Kurata puts people at ease right away. He rises above the petty tension that exists in most interactions between individuals. I visited him 3 times. Each time, I made an appointment, but then actually went to see him at a completely different time. The first time, I called just before going over, and he said "Just give me 10 minutes, and I'll be ready. I just got out of the shower, and don't have any clothes on." The unassuming, familiar tone in which he said this led me to respond "that's okay, I don't mind" – a very familiar, un-Japanese response.

I was so taken by Dr. Kurata's manner, and by the similarities between him and Mr. T., that I made up my mind to bring the two of them together. Therefore, without even thinking about the inconvenience it might cause Mr. T., who was extremely busy, I dragged him over to meet Dr. Kurata. I had pictures of each of them in my possession and, as I suspected, they looked somehow alike.

Before meeting Dr. Kurata for the first time, I had been extremely anxious, but by my second visit he had put me a wise old hermit." But, I thought, hermits are disconnected from reality. His reply only made me more anxious. I regretted asking.

In this way, my whale adventures had begun in Palau, brought me back to Japan, and were now taking me back once again to Palau. When I got back to Palau, I gave Mr. T. a report on how my research had been coming along. The truth was that I had learned almost nothing. Even so, Mr. T. just listened calmly.

Several days later, I went to meet Dr. Kurata. Dr. Kurata had graduated from the Palau South Seas Government's Fisheries College before World War II. At that time, Palau was administered by Japan, and Dr. Kurata, while working at the South Seas Government's Experimental Fisheries Station, was conscripted to fight in the battle of Angaur. During World War II, Palau was the scene of fierce fighting: between the battles of Peleliu and Angaur, approximately 15,000 Japanese and US soldiers lost their lives. After the war, Dr. Kurata worked at the Tokyo Experimental Fisheries Station, and then as the head of the Ogasawara Experimental Fisheries Center, and he was now living in Palau.

Dr. Kurata was extremely knowledgeable, had a very sharp mind, and was a logical thinker, so much so that he did indeed seem to be quite unlike other people. Perhaps this was why people talked about him being like a hermit, hallways were dark, and the rooms small, with books and documents stacked up everywhere so that there was no place to stand, specimens preserved in formaldehyde in glass jars all around. Dr. Yamada was talking earnestly to a young researcher.

I waited at the entrance until the professor interrupted his talk with the other researcher to usher me in. He told me a lot, but I got the impression that there was still much that wasn't known about whale migration routes. The professor said that the distribution charts that appeared in books should not be trusted, because they only noted "points" where whales that had been labeled had been spotted – they didn't show the whole picture.

Dr. Yamada showed me whale bones stacked floor to ceiling in a storeroom, and said that whale skeletons were his specialty and, since he didn't know too much about migration routes, he suggested I talk to Dr. Kurata on Palau and, on the spot, he contacted the organization with which Dr. Kurata was affiliated. I was again amazed, and grateful, to be treated with such kindness. (Or else, perhaps Dr. Sakurai had told Dr. Yamada what an odd character I was, and he did it just to humor me.)

Dr. Yamada said that Dr. Kurata was a very famous professor to whom all marine biology researchers were extremely indebted. People I didn't know made me nervous, though. I asked Dr. Yamada a lot of questions about what kind of a person Dr. Kurata was. (Was he approachable?) Dr. Yamada told me that "he's kind of like very town that was the setting for *Harpoon*, and C.W. Nicol himself had lived there for 1 year to gather information for the book. After talking about his research, Dr. Sakurai said to me: "Since whale migration routes are not my field of expertise, I am going to write you a letter of introduction to Dr. Yamada of the S Museum." I was amazed at the kindness he was showing to me, an amateur who didn't even work in the field, and who had just dropped in out of the blue. I was also amazed at the mysterious relationship binding people and whales together through the ages.

Right after returning home, I bought a copy of *Harpoon* from a used bookstore (it was unfortunately out of print, in both the English and Japanese editions, and I was only able to find it at a used book store). *Harpoon* is a story about traditional whaling; the protagonist is a young harpooner who has lost an arm to a shark. It is an epic historical novel set against the background of the upheaval of the Tokugawa shogunate era. Thanks to Dr. Sakurai, I was able to read again for the first time in a long time. I was really happy to have been able to rediscover the joy of reading.

I made an appointment with Dr. Yamada, and went to see him. He had a gentle smile, and his laboratory was the very picture of what I imagined the laboratory of a biologist specializing in field work should look like. The had already resigned from my position at the hospital, maybe I should cut back on work even more.

A while after I returned home from that trip, a whale became stranded on an island in Palau. Mr. T. contacted me and said he had a mission for me: to research how Palau was connected to whale migration routes. He said it would be good for me to get involved in something other than work for a change.

It sounded exciting to research whales, the largest mammal on earth; it also most definitely had nothing to do with psychiatry. However, I knew nothing about whales. So I went to my favorite bookstore, *SANSEIDO* in Jinbocho, and bought several books on whales. I learned a fair amount about the different whale species, but I couldn't find the information I was looking for about migration routes. In addition, I learned that some whale species migrated and some didn't. I decided it would be easier and faster to just ask a specialist in person, so I made an appointment with Dr. Sakurai, a curator at the W Museum, and went to visit him.

Dr. Sakurai told me that he had read C.W. Nicol's book *Harpoon* when he was in high school, and had become fascinated by traditional Japanese whaling techniques. He had done research in a museum on the east coast of the USA, and later became a curator at the W Museum after coming back to Japan. The W Museum was located in the

15

Whale Travels

I had been to Palau I don't know how many times, and I occasionally rode in the same boat with Mr. T., an underwater videographer. He was a professional videographer who produced films for television for many countries, including National Geographic specials shown in the USA, and he had a marvelous aesthetic sensibility. He had been making videos of guests, so I had him make a DVD for me, as well.

After I got home, I sent him a note thanking him for making me the DVD and saying how much fun it had been to go diving together. His reply surprised me. He signed it "Be strong." Normally, I would expect to see "Best regards" or "Warm regards" or something like that, but "Be strong"? I had not said anything about my private life to him, but he must have heard from one of the guides who had known me for a while that a close friend of mine had died.

The next time I met Mr. T., I told him about my clinical depression. That was unusual for me; normally, I never talk about my private affairs with others. However, because he was such a straightforward, honest person, I somehow felt confident that he wouldn't tell anybody about it. He was concerned, and said that, even though I transformed into something akin to marine snow, and float down and disappear into a miles-deep ocean trench.

I was staring down into the depths trying to verify this vision. If only I could look hard enough, I thought, surely I would be able to see myself breaking apart and sinking to the bottom.

Blue water is sometimes simply dark, and appears to have no bottom. There are also times when sunlight reaches down below the surface, and everything seems to sparkle with a bluish tint. When the ocean looks blue, and I gaze at it for a long time, I lose all sense of distance and clarity. There are times when I feel as if it continues out to infinity, and times when it seems as if there is a blue wall right next to me.

By going diving, I was trying to change my environment, to free myself from certain thoughts, and to somehow find the light at the end of the tunnel that was my clinical depression. However, it was more like a maze – the exit was not easy to find. Whenever I thought I could see it, it would turn out to be a mirage, and I would envision myself crouched over in the middle of a dark storm. Soon, I thought, I would probably stop believing that an exit even existed.

those days. My entries were all like this:

> "Date: MM / DD / YY
> Dive site: Blue Corner;
> Dive start time: 10:03; End time: 11:09;
> This dive: 1 hour 06 minutes;
> Maximum depth: 23.8 m;
> Average depth: 12.5 m;
> Water temperature: 28.2 degrees;
> Comments: (blank)."

Instead, I was busy looking down, into the invisible depths of the ocean. When I was a beginner, not being able to see the bottom of the deep ocean had made me nervous. When diving along a wall, I would be too scared to look down, and I would look only at the wall. Yet here I was just staring down into the bottomless depths.

When my symptoms were severe, I would be haunted by visions. One such vision was a vision of the deep, dark ocean. I would be in the middle of the dark ocean, slowly coming apart, bit by bit, into little pieces, which would disperse over a wide area of several kilometers and float silently to the bottom. In what is called the mid-deep zone of the ocean, where the ocean is several hundred meters deep, the world is completely dark – light does not reach down that far. In the middle of that darkness, I would break apart into countless nearly invisible particles,

Later, when I started to become mentally unbalanced, diving acted as a great stress reducer. Mr. Shimada, who had lots of experience both diving and free diving since his student days, told me that he had stayed away from diving for a long time after he started working, but that he had started diving again after his body started to fall apart from working too hard.

However, even diving, an activity that had initially been a stress reducer for me and that I had enjoyed so much, became impossible. Once, I made lodging and dive shop reservations but, as my scheduled departure date approached, I discovered that I didn't feel at all like going. Right up until the day before I was to leave, I vacillated: would I even be able to dive in my current state, or would it just take too much effort? Should I cancel? I ended up going, but I didn't enjoy it.

When we dove that time, a guide showed me the local spots, a lot of rare fish, extremely small fish called macros, schools of enormous fish, and other ocean life. However, I would just get annoyed when the guide tried to point things out to me. I couldn't have cared less what they were. That is why my log book for that trip is filled with statistical information about the dive, but the spaces for comments are completely blank. It was like a diary in which only the date, the weather, and the air temperature had been written down. I never described anything I saw; it was as if nothing important had happened on any of fins; schools of hundreds of barracuda or jacks; schools of sharks moving against a strong current simply by flexing their bodies ever so slightly: seeing such sights makes one forget all about life on land. Also, being carried along by powerful ocean currents make you realize just how weak and powerless you are. Your social status and material wealth on land vanish – in that moment, you come face to face with yourself simply as a human being.

Diving did indeed change my life. In fact, close friends I made through diving took care of me after I became depressed. Dr. Sakai and a mutual friend, Ms. Sera, took me out to eat, and even took me to Okinawa in order to get me a change of scenery. He kept telling me not to die on him. I once asked him why he was being so nice to me. He said that it was because we were fellow divers – and that was true, we had gone diving together twice. Mr. Shimada and Ms. Kanno, who had introduced me to diving, also took me out to dinner and called me often. Even though I was afraid of the phone, I would pick up when I heard their voices on the answering machine. I have no doubt that it must have been hard for them to call me up when they knew I might suddenly start crying in the middle of the conversation. They still called. To me, their support was like a life preserver to a drowning person.

I started diving about 2 years before I lost my first friend. At that time, I didn't have any signs of depression.

an unbelievable coincidence. Both encouraged me to definitely stick it out and get my C card and start diving. One of the drivers had even been a commercial diver, and he told me that "diving can change people's lives. I think it will change your life, too." I didn't think that there would be many things I could possibly do that had the potential to change my life, so I resolved on the spot to complete the classes and get my C card. Even though I am completely unathletic, and it therefore took me many times longer than most people to get the hang of it, once I made it past 100 dives, I started really enjoying being underwater.

Humans are land animals, held down to the earth by gravity, breathing air, and living in largely man-made surroundings. However, in the water, you don't have to walk. By inflating a BCD (buoyancy control device) jacket with air from your tank, or simply by adjusting your own breathing, you can move up and down as you like. You can then pick a spot and come face to face with truly natural, wild underwater animals, with nothing man-made in sight. The only problems are that you can't make it back to the surface without tank air and the currents can sometimes be quite strong. In other words, diving is accompanied by a degree of risk appropriate to any harsh natural environment.

Gorgeous, multicolored, coral reef fish; manta and eagle rays gracefully gliding through the water, fluttering their

14

Where Is the End of the Tunnel?

Since I resigned, I have gone diving in Palau several times. If you don't dive, you may not have heard of Palau, a republic encompassing more than 340 islands in Micronesia in the western Pacific Ocean that is about an hour and a half by plane from Guam.

My introduction to diving was fateful, in a way. I began diving at the urging of Mr. Shimada, a close friend, but I wasn't able to get my certification card, my "C card," on my first try. The instructor for my first diving course was a woman in her twenties who had just gotten her instructor's certificate. During a training dive in the ocean, I was caught in a rip current, and floated off with the instructor. Fortunately, two male instructors who had been watching us from the beach came to our rescue, but that incident scared me, and I dropped out of the course. However, I didn't want to give up, so I found another dive shop, explained what had happened, started taking classes again from the beginning, and got my C card.

The second time I tried to get my C card, both when I first when to the shop, and again one day on the way back from pool practice, I took taxis, and on both occasions I learned that the taxi drivers used to dive. This seemed like minds. Therefore, when their symptoms let up a little bit, they desperately want to conclude that they are finally on the road to recovery, and they immediately start trying to catch up on their backload of work. Or they test themselves to see how much they can accomplish. I used to regularly advise patients with clinical depression that they should only do half as much as they thought they could, but when it was my time to be depressed, I became completely incapable of making good decisions about such things. As soon as I would start to want to do things again, I would hastily conclude that I was almost back to normal, and that everything would be alright now, so I would throw myself headfirst back into my work. The result, of course, would be that afterwards I would be unable to get out of bed for several days in a row due to fatigue. Along with anxiety and irritability, I would start worrying that I was not getting any better. Just how long would I have to put up with this, anyway?

At such times, you mustn't push yourself. If you push, the waves of emotion will only push back harder. When the time comes, your clinical depression will lift – it is important that you have the patience to wait, to wait for time to pass, as it surely will.

weight. However, they do not lose and gain weight in the way that normal people do; whether they are eating or not eating, some people who are depressed have no conscious control over how much they eat. This happened to me, as well. In the course of about a month, I lost close to 5 kg and then, after several months had passed, I suddenly developed a tremendous appetite. Although it was extremely difficult, I made a conscious decision to leave food alone. But when I started actually trying to exercise conscious control over how much I ate, that only increased my stress level. I was able to lose a little weight again, but I don't know if that was because I had been successful in my efforts to leave food alone, or if my increased appetite had simply subsided.

Clinical depression prevents people from living their lives. They become unable to study, work, or clean their homes, and they blame themselves for these failings. They may be told by family members or friends that they are not being strict enough with themselves. However, even if they want to do something, they can't, because they don't have any energy. This is why you shouldn't try to push someone who is depressed to do anything. If you push them to try harder to do things, you will only push them away: it will make them feel as if they have no place left to go, no one to whom they can turn for support.

The fact that they are depressed and cannot fulfill their normal responsibilities is constantly preying on their then gripped by a nameless fear that something is going to get you, so you start to move. You want to scream. No matter how long you wait, the night never ends.

I had treated I don't know how many patients with extremely severe irritability (jitteriness), but even I hadn't imagined how bad it could actually be, that it would feel exactly as if one were being buffeted about by enormous waves in a fierce storm far out at sea.

Moreover, in the course of clinical depression, symptoms can emerge that are exact opposites of one other, separated by a certain interval of time, making you alternately lethargic and restless. There were times when I would have horrible, relentless insomnia, and then days when I would sleep for sixteen hours or more. Insomnia and hypersomnia, too little and too much sleep. While it is more normal for a person with clinical depression to have insomnia, there are certainly people who have hypersomnia, and also people who have both.

It is the same with food. While most people lose their appetite and become unable to eat, and therefore lose weight, some people start eating too much. Some people start wanting to eat incredible quantities of sweets: pastries, ice cream, chocolate, candy bars. When their clinical depression worsens, some people will lose their appetites, and so lose weight; then, when they start to get better, they will get their appetites back, and regain the who can pinpoint exactly when their condition got better or worse, like a light switch being turned on or off, the primary factors contributing to illness in such individuals, including people who become manic, are intrinsic – that is to say, biological. Such people are a minority.

There are also times in clinical depression when a person who has gotten over the worst of it and who has been getting better will temporarily get worse again: two steps forward, one step back. Such ups and downs are hard to bear, even when you expect them. It can feel just like being in the middle of a thunderstorm, being pushed this way and that by the wind, back and forth. William Styron, the Pulitzer Prize winning author I mentioned earlier, wrote that the English word "depression" does not accurately express the nature of this illness. He said that emotions can rage violently inside the brain, like a storm, and so the term "brain storm" would be more appropriate. I agree.

Another possible analogy would be wandering aimlessly through a dense forest at night in the middle of a storm, the lightning flashing, the thunder roaring, and the rain beating down in torrents. It is very cold, and dark. Trying in vain to find shelter, you huddle next to a large tree, but the cold rain runs down your back unmercifully. There are no roads, and you don't know which way to go to find shelter. You stay still and try not to move, thinking you will only exhaust yourself trying to escape, but are about what I would do if I started getting withdrawal symptoms. Fortunately, I never did. However, as soon as I had managed to somehow make it through the work day, with what little concentration I had left I would inevitably find myself wanting a glass of Champagne. At such times, I would make myself wait: I would say to myself "well, I won't drink today; I'll hold off until tomorrow and, if I still really want a drink, I'll think about it again then." In addition, Mr. T, who knew that I had stopped drinking, was constantly encouraging me to stay on the wagon.

It is not absolutely necessary to stop drinking if you are clinically depressed but, if you find yourself starting to drink more, you need to be careful.

13

The Rollercoaster

It is normal in clinical depression, even in patients who are making good progress, to have ups and downs. People's bodies are not machines – they do not run like clockwork. For example, just because overwork may have happened to be the trigger for the onset of clinical depression in a particular individual, that doesn't mean that person's condition will start to improve as soon as he or she takes some time off. While there are some people few days on which I had not had a drink. I would drink any type of alcohol, but Champagne, beer, and other fizzy drinks were my favorites. My decision to give up drinking was prompted by several unrelated incidents, the most significant of which was that, once I recognized that I was clinically depressed, I became scared that I would become dependent on alcohol. In truth, if I thought it would have helped me relax, even a little bit, I would have drunk however much it took. Since I had been working less after my resignation, it was not as if I couldn't take the next day off if I was hung over. However, that thought only scared me even more.

Through extensive clinical experience, I knew all too well how hard it is to treat alcohol abuse and dependence. It always horrified me the extent to which someone's personality would change due to alcohol-induced mental disorders, even though they themselves would not notice.

It is difficult to drink in moderation, to control how much you drink. This is even more true in clinical depression. If you really want to avoid getting an alcohol-induced disorder, the only sure way is to give up drinking. I had never drunk to the point where it had interfered with my day-to-day life, and although maybe I didn't really need to give it up completely, I decided that this would be a good time to do it. Although I didn't drink that much each day, I had been drinking for a long time, so I was very anxious for the first few days after quitting, worrying

12

On the Wagon

Although I did make several bad decisions, as described above, fortunately I was also able to do something that you would think should have given me some relief: I gave up drinking. People who regularly drink alcohol often drink more when they become depressed. In small quantities, alcohol alleviates tension and anxiety, and improves one's mood somewhat. Therefore, some people believe that drinking alcohol will help them relax, and they start drinking more and more. Pretty soon, they are drinking in the morning, as well, and end up becoming alcoholic.

When you drink too much alcohol, your sleep becomes shallower, your insomnia gets worse, and the hangovers weaken you physically, leaving you more and more fatigued. You also start blaming yourself for drinking so much. When you start drinking more, you think that it will help you escape from the harsh reality of your existence, but you are simply deluding yourself – your reality remains unchanged. On the contrary, it just means that you might end up with alcohol-induced liver damage to go along with your clinical depression.

I had been in the habit of having a drink with dinner for at least 10 years, during which time there had only been a only continue. This unfortunately caused me to turn my attention even more to my symptoms and my feelings of despair, in spite of the fact that I was trying at that time to maintain a certain distance from my symptoms, to view them more objectively, in order to avoid getting swept away by them.

Maybe that was just a coincidence, but these aggressive attempts by people to convert me to their religions only increased my fear and distrust of other people.

Religious people, when they see nonreligious friends fall upon hard times, think that their religion can save them and, with all the best intentions, recommend that they become believers, as well. However, as I said before, religion is fundamentally connected with one's outlook on life, and I don't think that a decision about whether to join a particular religion is one that can be made by someone who is suffering from clinical depression. If you are suffering from clinical depression, you may have friends recommend their religions to you, as well as many other things, but what you need to do is rest and seek treatment, not try out a bunch of new things.

However, one's religion is fundamentally related to one's outlook on life, and choosing a religion is a serious decision. I debated whether or not to join my friend's religion for more than a month.

I ultimately came to the conclusion that I would not be able to join. Even though my symptoms were so severe that I wanted to die, my feelings towards religion had not changed. I had known this friend for not a short time, and I felt extremely uncomfortable telling her of my decision. I blamed myself for allowing her to believe I might join, and then disappointing her, for letting it possibly become a source of friction between us and letting it get to the point where we might not be able to go back to the way we had been before, and for not decisively declining her invitation from the start. In addition, the stress of being pressured to make such a difficult decision, and the stress of the associated interactions with my friend, caused my symptoms to worsen considerably.

At virtually the same time, I was also asked by someone else from a different religion to join their religion. Apparently, this person had heard from someone who worked at a certain hospital that I had quit my job, and was worried about me. However, I didn't know who had spread this information about me – I hadn't even heard their name before, nor ever talked to them in person.

Both of these people told me that, if I didn't decide to join their religions as soon as possible, my suffering would

Since I had resigned for work reasons, in my case my clinical depression hadn't affected my decision to resign. However, apart from resigning from my job, the indecisiveness brought on by my clinical depression caused me to make several bad decisions. One of these was to decide to start work again at a new job. This was in spite of the fact that I was in no condition to go back to work. However, for various reasons, I ended up abandoning this plan at the last minute, greatly inconveniencing several people, and causing me to feel sorry for myself to boot.

Another bad decision involved an invitation from a friend to join her religion. I myself wasn't really a religious person. My friend knew that I was suffering, and told me that all her fellow believers were praying for me. She said that members of her religion would talk about people they knew who were in need of help, and then everyone would pray for them. They had all prayed for me, a complete stranger, and someone from outside their religion, at that. The next time I saw my friend, she urged me to join. Normally, at that point, had I not been depressed, I would have been able to explain my stance on religion clearly. However, by that point I had already been depressed for a long time, and I was desperate, and willing to try anything to rid myself of the pain, so I gave a noncommittal response.

passed.

There was nothing I could do to prevent these feelings from welling up inside me – it would just happen. Sometimes they would sneak up on me, and sometimes they would hit me all at once, like a bolt from the blue. However, when I would get these feelings, I would try to remind myself that this was my depression talking, that these were not my normal thoughts. I tried to look at myself more objectively, as if observing myself from a distance. When I did that, I became a little less afraid of being sucked down into the maelstrom of my own emotions.

11

Making Bad Decisions

When you are clinically depressed, it is hard to make all kinds of decisions. It takes more time and, even after you have made a decision, you worry endlessly that it was the wrong one. And since you are more pessimistic than normal, you are completely incapable of making decisions about important things. Until your clinical depression passes, it is impossible to make decisions about critical personal issues, such as marriage, divorce, retirement, moving, and so on, without regretting them later.

counted how many tablets I had. Then I went back to the sofa and sat there some more.

My cat then came in from my bed, where she had been sleeping, and jumped up on the sofa and looked up at me. I looked back. She is a silver tabby with a beautiful coat and pretty green eyes. She just sat there and stared at me. I stared back. To a cat, being looked at directly signals an impending attack. Even so, she didn't look away. She just sat there, unmoving. I stroked her face. Her fur was soft and supple.

She just stared at me like that for what seemed like a very long time. I eventually reassured her that I was okay: "it's alright," I whispered, in a voice so quiet I could barely hear myself.

I thought that well, at any rate, I could wait until tomorrow to die. I thought that, even if I were going to die, I wasn't going to kill myself in my own home. I wasn't going to kill myself in front of my cat, and I couldn't die until I found someone to take care of her. She sat with me on the sofa until I got up and went back to bed.

In truth, there had been many times when I had been thinking of ways to die. That night was just the time when I felt most compelled to do it. Although that was the only time it really seemed as if I might actually go through with it, my feelings of wanting to die were always present, although in varying levels of intensity. I would try to somehow not let them bother me, and to wait until they diver, through the shredder. Log books, as the name indicates, are records of all the dives a diver has made. The date, time, location, and site of each dive, the tank pressure before and after the dive, water temperature, maximum depth, average depth, visibility, life-forms seen, comments of fellow divers, and so on – one's entire diving history. I had held off for a long time on getting rid of my log books, but in the end, I got rid of them, too (except for the most recent one).

Then, my insomnia got really bad. I couldn't sleep. I would listen to the sounds of the trains going by in the otherwise silent night outside my window. The sounds of the trains would stay with me for hours on end, and when they would finally fall silent, I would know that the last train of the night had gone by. Then, sleep would finally come … or so I would think, but then I would awaken with a start after only a few hours, at around 2 or 3 in the morning. I would be wide awake, almost eerily so and, once awake, I would get intensely jittery, and couldn't remain lying down.

After several nights like that, one night, when I woke up, I was seized a terrible restlessness. I got up, went into the living room, turned on the light, and sat there on the sofa for a while.

I felt like I couldn't take it anymore. I went into the kitchen, opened the drawer of my medicine chest, and that I felt duty-bound to accomplish, although I hadn't expected to be doing it under these circumstances. My friend had asked me, on a number of occasions, "if I die, please do this for me," and I was busy concentrating on getting it done.

My friend's request was not easily accomplished. It took several months, and required the help of the people who had been his closest friends while he was alive. When it was finished, I suddenly found myself deeply unsettled.

I reached a crisis point around the beginning of the summer. I became more and more restless, and could not sit still or even stay home. I couldn't sleep. I tried to kill time, but I couldn't even read, one of my favorite pastimes, because I couldn't concentrate. So I would wander around town for hours, and would then be too tired to get out of bed the next day.

I started getting rid of personal items, mementos, and things I didn't need. I threw away a lot of stuff. A part of me didn't want to, but another part of me didn't want to leave anything behind if something were to happen, and that part of me won out. After I would get rid of something, I would feel pleased with myself – I would be glad I had done it. I threw away all my old letters and photos.

In addition to reading, I liked scuba diving, but I even put my log books, records which are very important to a

There were many places in the world where people were suffering under horrible conditions, where people were dying every day, and here I was, leading a good-for-nothing life, surrounded by privilege. If there was someone else who wanted my life, I thought, they could have it. There was nothing I wanted to do. I had lost all hope, all desire.

Thoughts that would have never even occurred to me before, when I was healthy, swirled inside my head. I had finally reached the point where I honestly couldn't do anything, anything at all.

People can continue living as long as they have even one goal or hope. But I had absolutely none; this must have been what William Styron meant by "the despair beyond despair."

10

Wanting to Die

Several days after my second close friend died, a colleague, Dr. Sakai, called and told me that everyone was worried that I might kill myself. I wondered why they would think that. In fact, I was preoccupied with a task myself, I had occasionally been depressed and felt like crying, but I had wondered whether or not there were really full-grown adults who cry or "talk tearfully" that much. Unfortunately, I came to realize firsthand that the diagnostic criteria and symptom evaluation scales for clinical depression capture a more accurate picture of depression than I had originally thought.

9

Being Pessimistic

Along with suddenly feeling like crying for no reason, I gradually became more and more pessimistic. I started to wonder why I had been able to become a psychiatrist even though I had no talent. I started thinking that I wouldn't be able to work again, and that I wouldn't be able to support myself financially.

I started blaming myself for things that had happened in the past, and also for random, abstract events. I wondered why I was alive, and what a waste of time and energy my whole life had been. I started thinking that every single choice I had ever made in my life had been a mistake, but that I couldn't take any of them back. And I started thinking that my family would have been much happier if I had never been born.

depressed in the normal sense of the word, it is fair to say that the depression experienced by healthy individuals in the course of their daily lives is completely different in content and severity from that experienced by people with clinical depression.

For example, in the first moments after opening my eyes in the morning, I would feel indescribably bad - some unidentifiable combination of great sadness and intense anxiety. I would wonder if I could tolerate living through one more whole day. I would wonder: Why did I have to open my eyes? Wouldn't it have been so much better if I could have just left my eyes closed forever. On work days, I would eventually muster up the strength to get out of bed, wash my face, take a shower, and leave home. Then, on my walk to the station, I would suddenly feel tears welling up inside me, for no reason. I wouldn't be crying, exactly, it would be more like something building up inside my chest, inside my eyes. I would feel as if I were suffocating, and have chest pains. These feelings would come upon me in waves, unbidden, and were extremely distressing. It would be all I could do to keep from crying on my walk to the station. The air would feel heavy, and I would barely have enough energy to breathe.

One rating scale that is commonly used to evaluate depression includes the categories "crying" and "talking tearfully." Before I experienced clinical depression for

8

Being Clinically Depressed

In addition to not having any energy in the morning, there were times when I thought "now that I think about it … isn't that a symptom of clinical depression." The most characteristic symptom of clinical depression is depressed mood ("depression" in laymen's terms). However, it is extremely common for depressed individuals to not be aware of their own depressed moods. Even when they come in to the doctor's office with a clear lack of energy and a pained expression, sometimes even crying, they will say "I'm not really depressed." Some people feel anxious or irritable more than they feel depressed. In addition, clinical depression can manifest itself in many different ways: "I don't have any energy," "nothing is fun for me," "I feel pessimistic," "I feel like I have no future," "I feel nothing but despair," "I feel like crying."

William Styron, a journalist who won a Pulitzer Prize and went on to become an author, became clinically depressed and was hospitalized in a psychiatric hospital. He wrote about his struggle with clinical depression in a book titled "*Darkness Visible*," in which he states that clinical depression is "the despair beyond despair."

While there is probably no one who has never felt

known that the symptoms of clinical depression fluctuate during the day, and it is often the case that the symptoms will be more severe in the morning and then milder in the afternoon and evening. Of course, for some people the whole day is bad, and for some people the evenings are worse, but feeling worse in the morning is a characteristic symptom of clinical depression. When I noticed that I couldn't concentrate and had no energy in the morning, but would start feeling better in the afternoon, it hit me with a shock that this was a classic feature of clinical depression.

I realized all over again that my depression had deteriorated to the point where it was interfering with my normal functioning, so much so that I was going to have to quit my job. Then, even after I quit and was working only part-time, my depression continued preventing me from functioning normally. It was clear that I was experiencing not just a temporary condition, like the "blues" that everyone gets from time to time, but was, in fact, suffering from clinical depression, a psychiatric disorder. I finally had to stop kidding myself that I wasn't clinically depressed.

about 100 papers in order to write a review of the topic I had been given. However, academic papers use a standard format: every single one is laid out the same, with an introduction, an explanation of the subject of the research, an explanation of the study method, a description of the results, and discussion and conclusions sections, in that order. Once you're used to them, they're not that hard to read. Also, at the very beginning there is a short passage called an "abstract" that summarizes the entire paper.

However, when I would sit down in front of that pile of papers and pick one up, I couldn't muster up the interest to read it. When I would try to will myself to read it anyway, I would only manage to get through a few lines before I couldn't go on. I couldn't even make it through the short abstract at the beginning and, what was worse, I couldn't follow what it was talking about at all, and I had to read the same lines over and over again. I felt like my brain was completely nonfunctional. Even though the deadline for submitting the review had already passed, I abandoned all work on it for another good two weeks. The time flew by. Every day I would see the pile of unread papers, and my blank computer screen – the only thing I had typed was the title.

I struggled to somehow make progress on it. I first looked through the titles of the papers and categorized them by subject. I found that, in the morning, I couldn't muster up any energy to work on them but that, in the afternoon, I would be able to read a little bit. It is well other specialties at several different hospitals. The mind and body are closely linked.

7

Becoming Aware of Your Depression

Individuals with mental illnesses often cannot bring themselves to accept that they have a problem. Clinical depression is no exception. Recognizing that you yourself are ill is referred to as "insight of disease," and I did not gain this until several months after I had resigned from my job.

Even though I had resigned, I still had piles of work that I had not finished, as well as papers I had been asked to write. Besides, it was not as if I had enough savings to just quit working completely. I was also scared that once I stopped working I wouldn't be able to start again. And, like a racehorse running a race, I thought I couldn't just come to a sudden stop right at the finish line – I needed to cool down . I decided to work part-time, 4 days a week, at institutions other than the one I had left.

The first thing I had to do was to prepare a manuscript with a fast approaching deadline. I had to read at least been really tough, it being a Tuesday and all. The four of them just looked at me and said nothing. There was silence. Then, the doctor finally said: "It's Friday."

I froze. Normally, I'm never wrong about the day.

In that instant, I realized that, in my mind, the only thing that existed was the present – right now – the past and the future didn't exist for me. The day of the week, the date, the month, the year, none of it meant anything to me.

The two nurses started saying that they wanted me to stay at my job, but I wasn't really listening. Sitting there in that restaurant, talking and eating, was unbearable. After I got home, I just stood there in the middle of the room, paralyzed by fear, sure that this was the onset of dementia.

When people are clinically depressed, they sometimes start worrying that maybe they have come down with some kind of serious physical illness. Put another way, when people are depressed, they often experience physical symptoms. Clinical depression is not just a disorder of mood or willpower. Decreased appetite, headaches, constipation, dry mouth, palpitations, lethargy, and many other physical symptoms emerge. For this reason, sometimes people don't recognize their problem as clinical depression right away, and are only referred to a psychiatrist after having been examined by doctors in offered to refer me to an acquaintance. However, that would have meant remaining in the United States for several months, and it hardly seemed likely that I would be up to the task of preparing for such a journey.

Furthermore, even at this stage I still didn't want to admit that I was depressed. I felt like I couldn't tolerate that in myself. It took until several months after I had resigned before I finally had to acknowledge to myself that I was clinically depressed.

Although I myself was never treated by a specialist, this is unusual, and absolutely should be avoided. I most likely would have gotten better more quickly had I been properly treated.

6

Am I Physically Ill?

When I resigned from my position at the hospital, a few of the younger doctors and nurses said that they would like to take me out to dinner. On the day in question, the five of us were to go to an Italian restaurant. I and the two nurses took my car, and we made it to the restaurant on time, as did one of the doctors. The other doctor was late, having just come from another hospital. When he sat down, I casually mentioned that office hours must have

There was a reason why I continued avoiding going to a specialist. If you are a psychiatrist, you use both medication and psychotherapy to treat clinical depression, no matter who the patient. In addition to finding out whether or not there are any psychological triggers for the depression, if patients are under any psychological stress, it is normal to try to find ways of helping them deal with it. In my case, stress from both my professional and private lives had served as the triggers for the onset of my depression. I had a lot of information, such as confidential work information, that I wasn't supposed to talk about with anyone. However, I couldn't shake the feeling that, if I went to therapy and was asked, nicely and kindly, I would start talking about things I shouldn't, or mustn't, talk about. Since the psychiatrist who would be treating me would also have a confidentiality obligation, while theoretically we should be able to talk freely about anything, I became gripped by fear, and started feeling as if I could trust none of my colleagues. I also didn't want my personal issues to be recorded in such detail. Furthermore, if I ended up being examined at a clinic or, worse, a hospital, there was the chance I might run into a psychiatrist other than the one treating me. Any of the staff seeing my insurance card would know where I worked.

Dr. D, an English psysician who had seen how depressed I was, suggested I seek treatment in the United States, and conditions were unstable took more and more time, and I was constantly worrying that I had made a mistake.

Eventually, I became so depressed that I had to quit – in other words, it got to the point where I couldn't get on with my life. Some people kindly suggested that maybe I should just take some time off, but I myself couldn't accept that from someone in my position, even if it would only be for a short time.

5

Seeking Treatment

I decided that I would resign at the end of the academic year. I would use paid vacation to take some time off but, even so, I wasn't confident that I would be able to make it to the end of the year. At that point, I should have seen a psychiatrist and started receiving expert care. But, after all, I was a psychiatrist myself, wasn't I? Who in the world could I ask to treat me? I finally asked Dr. Sakai, a more senior doctor, to prepare for me, as a friend, a medical certificate in case I would have to take time off from work. He was kind enough to prepare it for me, even though I ended up never using it.

afraid that I wouldn't know who it was, or that it would be someone bringing bad news, or that I would be uncomfortable not being able to see the face of the person on the other end of the line, or that I wouldn't be able to understand what they were talking about, or that I would start crying in the middle of the conversation. I could no longer answer the phone. I would let the answering machine pick up, and just sit there, staring blankly, and listen. I couldn't even watch television any longer. The news was particularly stressful, with reports every day about terrorism, cruelty, and natural disasters. Seeing those images only heightened my anxiety and made by heart beat faster.

Corresponding with people via e-mail became difficult, as well, and it became extremely hard for me to work. If I got an e-mail that was too long or complicated, I wouldn't have the energy to read it through to the end. I couldn't understand what it was saying, either. And responding was out of the question. I honestly became incapable of reading or responding to any e-mail more than five lines long. Because I had to, I would take care of my business by making telephone calls, but that required a tremendous amount of effort.

Amazingly, even in this state, I continued to treat patients. Actually, existing patients who were stable were no problem, but examining new patients or patients whose this alternate reality. It reminded me of the story "Dream of the Butterfly," an old Chinese tale about a monk who dreams he is a butterfly and then, upon waking, thinks: am I a man who dreamed he was a butterfly, or a butterfly dreaming he is a man. Which is the true reality? Everything seemed unreal. I felt as if my mind had left my body and were floating, detached, a few feet away. This is actually a common symptom of clinical depression that is called "depersonalization."

My friend had died on a Wednesday so, every Wednesday morning, I would be seized by a terrible feeling of dread. I would be afraid that I would get a telephone call reminding me of the death of my friend, and that my entire breakdown would start all over again, from the beginning. It was unbearable. My memory started failing me. I had always been able to remember exactly who I had met, and when, and what we had talked about but now, for the life of me, I couldn't remember anything like that at all. Even events that had happened only yesterday, or the day before, became lost in a kind of fog, and I became deeply worried that this forgetfulness was in fact the beginnings of dementia. I couldn't even remember appointments I had made with people, and I had to start writing them down in my notebook.

It became very stressful for me to simply meet or talk with other people. I was terrified of the phone. I was insecurity; I fell into a slump. I had hit a wall that I couldn't seem to get over, and I approached one of the senior teaching doctors for advice. The instructor, who was a top anesthesiologist, said to me "You're not the type of person who gets over barriers; you're the type who smashes through them. You? In a 'slump?' You must be joking!" I was not the type of person who normally talked to others about my private issues, so I probably hadn't made it as clear as I should have that I was really suffering and needed real help, not simply light-hearted words of encouragement. At any rate, while I may have seemed powerful, the type to smash through barriers, to my colleague, in truth I was powerless.

Then, the shock of my second close friend dying in the spring of the following year was the final blow. It was just too sudden. The shock of two such close friends dying two years in a row was too much for me. I knew that I had reached my limit. I could no longer continue on like this; something had to change.

A strange sensation came over me. I started feeling like I had somehow been transported to a different world. I starting feeling as if several worlds existed simultaneously in parallel universes, and that the world I was on now was not the real world at all but that, in the real world, wherever that was, my friends were still alive and I, through my own fault, had somehow gotten lost here, in on and off is meaningless. You mustn't just stop taking it on your own, and you must talk to your doctor about its effectiveness and side effects.

4

Reduced Quality of Life

The year that my first friend died, once the busy conference season had passed, my mood sank even lower than before, even though I had already started taking my first antidepressant drug. My personal treatment policies, as a doctor, had been in conflict on numerous occasions with the new administrative guidelines that had been instituted at my hospital, and this had demotivated me with respect to my job. In the bureaucracy of a large hospital, one person's objections simply go unheard. I felt that, if I couldn't abide by the rules of the organization, I had no choice but to resign. In addition, personal issues that had been bothering me for many years had recently become even more troublesome. The realization that I could not solve any of these problems was painful, and left me completely drained.

Having been insecure ever since I was a resident about my competence as a doctor, I finally fell victim to my antidepressant medications are about this effective, a level of effectiveness that is nevertheless demonstrably superior to that obtained from taking a placebo (a sugar pill). All antidepressants (and, in fact, not just antidepressants, but all medications) have intended, beneficial effects and unintended, adverse side effects that have been scientifically verified through clinical trials. If a medication has an effective rate of 50 to 70%, and a patient takes that medication and he or she gets better, then that person will undoubtedly feel that the medication is 100% effective. The problem is that it is impossible to know in advance who will be in this group of 50 to 70. It's simply a matter of trial and error; the only thing that can be done is to first try those drugs that seem as if they might be the most effective, based on the patient's symptoms, age, medical history, and physical complications. Therefore, just because I took one particular drug and it worked for me doesn't mean that it will work for you. Conversely, there are some people who could take several times as much of the drug that I couldn't take in sufficient doses because of the side effects, and who would get relief from that drug, and without any side effects.

What is important to remember if you are going to take an antidepressant is that it will take some time before it starts to work, and that you need to continue taking the prescribed dose in the prescribed manner, because taking it that maybe I was no longer really clinical depressed, that maybe the symptoms that remained were just side effects of the medication, and that I would get better if I would only stop taking the medication.

I got worse. My depressive moods, anxiety, irritability, and lack of energy all got worse. I needed to start taking medication again. Since I had not been able to use a high enough dose, and since I had been having side effects, I started taking a different medication. After several days, my irritability and anxiety disappeared completely. I could hardly believe it – on the days I didn't work, I was now able to just relax all day at home. Although my energy and concentration had not completely returned, and I sometimes felt like I was getting worse again, the new medication seemed to be better than the first at alleviating my symptoms.

For reasons I will explain later, I have decided not to identify the antidepressant medications that I took. There are several different classes of antidepressant medications, and many different drugs in each class, but which one will work varies depending on the individual. The probability of any one antidepressant medication being effective in a given individual is about 50 to 70%. This means that, if 100 patients take a given drug, from 50 to 70 of them will experience an improvement in their symptoms. Although these figures may lead some of you to think that these medications are not that effective, the fact is that all

I continued taking my medication, but I was not able to continue taking it until my symptoms started to improve, because the side effects had become too severe. Normally, patients are already fairly severely clinically depressed when they start taking medication, so they are willing to put up with the side effects to a certain extent for the sake of getting better. Later, as they start to get better, they notice their symptoms less, and the side effects more.

After about 6 months had passed since I started taking the medication, I was sick of taking so much medication, and I took this to mean that the reason I was noticing the side effects more was because I was getting better. I therefore stopped taking my medication. Unfortunately, that was a big mistake. About 1 or 2 weeks later, all my energy simply disappeared; I was unspeakably fatigued. Even though it had not cured me completely, clearly the antidepressant medication had been working.

It is said that you need to continue taking antidepressant medication for about 4 to 6 months after it starts working. If you stop taking the medication too soon, you suffer a relapse (your symptoms come back). Since I had stopped taking the medication before I had gotten well enough, I got worse again. The problem was that by the time I had stopped, my symptoms had already been waxing and waning for some time, and I had just become really sick of the whole idea of being on medication. I started thinking own to stop taking their medication if they start experiencing side effects, without even taking the time to tell their doctor. That is why it is particularly important for the doctor to ask about the effectiveness and side effects of any antidepressant medication soon after the patient starts taking it. Alternatively, family members or friends can accompany the patient to the doctor's office and tell the doctor about the side effects that the patient has been experiencing.

After I decided that I needed medication, I chose one that doesn't have such potent side effects and that starts working fairly quickly. For several days after I started taking it, I felt slightly nauseous, but not so much so that I couldn't deal with it. After about 2 weeks, some of my energy returned. I felt that the medication was starting to work, and I was somewhat relieved. I thought that, if I could just get through the peak conference season in the autumn, my workload would lighten up a bit, and maybe I would be alright. I had taken on a simply ridiculous amount of work that year. I had literally several times my normal workload. I didn't take my condition seriously enough. Since I wouldn't rest, any improvement or relief would be fleeting – I would squander my energy, and be worse again. I tried increasing my dosage in order to get through it somehow, but I wasn't able to increase it enough due to side effects: I experienced terrible, intolerable dizziness and nausea.

no identifiable cause, clinical depression needs to be treated. All the textbooks and manuals say that rest and treatment with antidepressant medication are both essential – like the two wheels of a bicycle. However, equally important is the support that one receives from one's inner circle of family and friends, but I still did not realize that. I learned that only several months after I had become unable to work. But I'm getting ahead of myself; let me return to the topic of antidepressants.

There are several different types of antidepressants. Since antidepressant medications had become my specialty, I had tried several different ones myself, not because I had been depressed, but in order to experience their side effects firsthand, so that I would be able to more easily empathize with what my patients were going through, and know what questions to ask them.

It takes a little time before antidepressants start working, at least several days to a week, and sometimes nearly a month. Side effects may or may not occur, depending on the dose and also on the individual. When they do occur, it tends to be in the first several days after starting the medication. Therefore, when taking an antidepressant, it is necessary to put up with the side effects while waiting for the medication to start working against the depression. Patients who are depressed and have no energy, for whom even carrying on a conversation requires tremendous effort, may simply decide on their colleagues, and about the meetings and appointments I would miss, and about how that would simply mean that I would have that much more work to do when I did end up going back to work, I would feel stress just thinking about calling up to take the day off. Inevitably, I would muster up the courage to go to work, but after I would get out of bed, I would then just sit right down again on the floor in front of my closet and not move, because I couldn't decide what to wear. It would take all my energy just to wash my face, and even then I would have to lean against the sink for support.

By nature, I am an early riser. I used to get to work early every day, but now I found myself coming to work later and later. I was never "late," per se, but the mornings were very hard. Even though my fighting with myself every morning about whether or not to go to work continued for several weeks, I myself, a specialist in mental disorders, did not even begin to suspect the truth about why I felt so awful in the morning: I was depressed.

3

Antidepressant Therapy

At any rate, I had to do something. Even when there is

At that time, I could still get to sleep, but when I would get up in the morning, I would be indescribably tired. Even though, having slept, I should have felt at least a little rested, I would somehow feel more tired than when I had gone to bed. I would think that there was no way I could go to work. I would lie in bed and fight with myself for what would seem like forever over whether or not to call in sick. I would go over and over all the possible excuses in my head: "I don't feel well"; "I have a fever"; "I've been feeling a little dizzy this morning"; "I've caught a bad cold." None of them would sound convincing. Everyone knew that I wasn't the type to not come in to work for something minor like that. I had been trained to believe that it was unacceptable to miss work for anything less than something like a broken leg; I had only missed about 5 days of work in the past 20 years. When you're working at a hospital, you can't just work hard for a little while, and then slack off. You need to show constant effort and dedication, and keep yourself in shape both physically and mentally. And, of course, you have to work as many hours as possible.

Even in the state I was in then, somehow I knew, albeit dimly, that one day off was not going to be enough to get my energy level back to normal. I knew that if I took one day off, it wouldn't stop there – I would probably end up taking several days off. When I started to think about how much me taking time off would inconvenience my happened, I never would have had to see a psychiatrist" – there are also times when there is no clear triggering event. In my case, the death of close friends acted as the twin triggers that set off my clinical depression. Their deaths occurred over a span of two years, and they were sudden, so there had been no time for me to prepare myself mentally. The death of the second friend really hit me hard but, by that time, which was about 1 year after the death of the first friend, I was already in what could be described as the initial stages of clinical depression. At that time, I was involved in educational and research activities at a certain research institution, and working as a teaching doctor at that institution's health care facility.

In the year that I lost my first friend, who died in April, I had taken on a lot of new responsibilities at work, and I was extremely tired. Every night, when I would get home from work, I wouldn't have the energy to say even one more word, and certainly not the energy to make dinner, so I would buy a sandwich at a deli close to my house. Since even choosing what to eat was a chore, I got the same combination sandwich every day: half ham and cheese on whole wheat, half egg salad on white. I would go home, drink a beer, eat a little of the sandwich and, since I would then be unable to get up, just lie down right there on the carpet. I would have to rest for just a little bit before I could muster up the energy to change my clothes, wash my face, and get into bed.

clinically depressed themselves to know what it was like. When you are in such agony, you feel that there is no way that you will ever get better. If only there were people who could step in for patients and explain to everyone in their lives what they are going through, what a tremendous help that would be. And, if those people could also explain to the patients themselves the nature of the symptoms that have consumed them so totally and unexpectedly, what tremendous comfort that would bring. It occurred to me that psychiatrists who have experienced depression themselves could be such people.

This is the true story of the clinical depression that I, a psychiatrist, experienced. I have written this book not for personal catharsis, but in the hope that it may serve as a useful reference explaining the true nature of clinical depression. Although I have altered some of the details slightly, the following descriptions of depression are based on my own real-life experience.

2

Triggers

Although there is sometimes a clear cause or trigger for the onset of clinical depression – "if only that had not crept unbidden back into my mind.

Even though I had been working as a psychiatrist for a long time, treating many patients for clinical depression the whole while, I realized that I hadn't understood it at all. The suffering I had been enduring over the past several months was surely payback for my ignorance. I felt as if I were being tortured for my foolishness. On top of that, I was now horrendously fatigued, my thoughts had slowed to a crawl, and I was wondering what on earth I was going to do – I had a 3-hour lecture to give soon, and it just didn't seem as if I was going to be able to pull it off. I almost wanted the plane to just crash.

However, at the same time, another part of me felt admiration for my patients for being able to overcome such feelings because, if they could cause me such pain even though I, a psychiatrist, was so knowledgeable about the symptoms and course of clinical depression, and should therefore have been more easily able to anticipate them, then how much more anxiety they must cause my patients, who had no such expert knowledge. I was impressed by the fact that people could hold up under such trying circumstances. Clinical depression is sometimes explained as being simply a more severe form of the depressed moods everyone experiences from time to time, but in fact it is completely different. Now, I finally understood why it was virtually impossible for family members, friends, or coworkers who had never been

1

Reminiscences at 35,000 Feet

"I don't know about me becoming a psychiatrist …."

Those had been my own words, spoken so long ago, back when I was a med student, sitting in a cramped, windowless room on the medical school campus.

"I don't think I'm really cut out for it," I had continued. "I think it's interesting as a field of study, but I personally have had a pretty easy life so far. I haven't gone through any really tough times myself, so I think I would probably have a hard time understanding what my patients are going through."

The counselor sitting across from me pointed out that, for one thing, I wasn't required to experience my patients' pain in order to be a psychiatrist and that, at any rate, he suspected that perhaps we wouldn't even be having this conversation if I had really had such an easy life as I made it sound.

It was late, and probably dark outside. My counseling session was over, and it was time for me to leave.

In the end, I did become a psychiatrist. Twenty years later, sitting on an airplane on my way to give a lecture, the memory of that conversation in that cramped, dreary room, a memory that had lain undisturbed for so long,

16 Trusting People 54
17 One Morning 55
18 Laughter 62
19 Someone to Lean On 68
20 Epilogue 71
   ❏

Reflections   **Mark Thorpe** 75

The Lost Phoenix   **Yoji Kurata** 81

About the translator 85

Underwater Images   **Mark Thorpe** 86

CONTENTS

Acknowledgements v
Preface ix
To the Person Holding This Book xiv

1 Reminiscences at 35,000 Feet 1
2 Triggers 3
3 Antidepressant Therapy 6
4 Reduced Quality of Life 12
5 Seeking Treatment 16
6 Am I Physically Ill? 18
7 Becoming Aware of Your Depression 20
8 Being Clinically Depressed 23
9 Being Pessimistic 25
10 Wanting to Die 26
11 Making Bad Decisions 30
12 On the Wagon 34
13 The Rollercoaster 36
14 Where Is the End of the Tunnel? 41
15 Whale Travels 47

for your interest. Clinical depression is an extremely common illness. Whether or not you yourself have ever actually been clinically depressed, it is an illness that can strike anyone. I hope that you will take this opportunity to learn a little bit about clinical depression and in the process perhaps lose some of your preconceptions about mental illness (if you have any).

way through, and they are not being lazy. This is one of the symptoms of clinical depression, and one of the reasons they need care.

- Although people often recover from clinical depression with only a few months of treatment, sometimes more time is required. Although it is certainly tough to stand by and watch as the time drags on, please try to avoid becoming impatient.

- People who are clinically depressed often become irritable and cranky. They may take it out on you, and say things to hurt you. However, they do not act like this when they are healthy, do they? Please stay calm – do not let yourself get caught up in their illness.

If you are neither clinically depressed nor a family member or friend of someone who is:

- Why did you pick up this book? Perhaps you are thinking that you might be depressed? If so, please do see a doctor. Seeing a psychiatrist or psychologist is nothing to be ashamed of. For example, would you think twice about going to the hospital if you had severe stomach pain?

- If you picked up this book simply because you are interested the topic of clinical depression, thank you

If you are a family member or friend of someone who is clinically depressed:

- Please educate yourself about the symptoms of clinical depression. The symptoms described in this book are relatively typical symptoms of clinical depression, but their severity will vary depending on the individual. Once a particular symptom becomes too severe, it may, conversely, become more difficult for the patient to complain about it or even to recognize it for what it is. Please pay attention to the patient's words and actions, and discuss any concerns you have with them and find out if they are suffering. Also, if it seems that they are not capable of adequately explaining their symptoms or the effectiveness or side effects of their medication to their doctor, go with them to their doctor and talk to the doctor yourself.

- If they start worrying that they are never going to get better, please remind them, over and over, that people always recover from clinical depression. Tell them not to panic, but to simply continue to rest and receive treatment.

- When they can no longer do things that they could do when they were not depressed, please don't try to encourage or push them to do anything. Clinical depression is not something that they can fight their

To the Person Holding This Book

This book does not discuss clinical depression from a medical perspective. Rather, the aim of this book is to give the reader a better understanding of clinical depression by telling the story of one individual, to show that recovery from depression is indeed possible.

If you have been diagnosed with depression:

- Do not try to force yourself to read this. If you feel yourself getting tired after reading just a few lines, or if you feel you just do not have the energy, put this book down, wait a few weeks, and then try again.

- Right now, you may feel that life is nothing but suffering; however, you must not choose death, for your condition will most assuredly change for the better. Have you told your doctor or people close to you about your difficulties? If not, do so, and ask for their help. Please do not hesitate to ask for help when you are suffering. If you do, you will find, perhaps to your surprise, that there are people you can turn to for support.

reason, the first half of my story may seem a little more disjointed, pessimistic, and emotionally barren than the second half. In the second half, I was more hopeful, and I started paying more attention to the flow of the story, I think. I have purposely avoided going back and revising the first half of the story to make it easier to read, however, since I think that the way the story was written in and of itself reflects the "thinking disturbance" (a symptom of depression) from which I was suffering at that time, and I hope that this may provide the reader with some additional insight into the nature of the disease.

Now then, allow me to be your guide on a tour of the maze of depression. Don't worry, though, with me as your guide, you will be able to find the exit.

Akemi

emerge from the dark maze of my depression. It has been a little more than a year since that time, and I have started a new job, made new friends, and am somehow continuing to live my life.

I still feel somehow uncertain even of my own existence, and I am sometimes beset by unwanted doubts about why I am alive, about the reason for my existence. However, I have also gained some valuable wisdom: if I had not experienced depression, I would not have come into contact with some truly wonderful people, and I would not understand and appreciate life the way I do now.

My editor, Ms. Sone, told me that my story would be easier to read if I could recall more conversations, and include them in the story. However, even though I tried hard for many days to recall at least a few conversations, I couldn't. When I was ill, it was extremely difficult to talk to people, and I often couldn't follow what they were saying, nor later remember what had been said. A storm had been raging inside of me, and I had been spending all of my energy trying to curl up into a ball, to withdraw into myself, for protection.

I started writing this story after I left my previous job, but while my condition was still unstable, and before I switched to a different antidepressant medication. For that caused my condition to take a sharp turn for the worse. Eventually, I was not able to continue working.

I left my job and started working on a part-time basis, but even then I did not get better. I thought that maybe I had been misinterpreting side effects of the drug I had been taking as symptoms of my depression, so I stopped taking my medicine - another mistake. I had already become unable to think things through logically and objectively. When I stopped taking my medication, my condition worsened, and only then did I appreciate how effective the medicine had been. Although this experience led me to conclude that I did, in fact, need drug therapy, I somehow couldn't bring myself to start taking the same drug again, because of its side effects. I tried switching to a different antidepressant. Although my symptoms improved somewhat after the switch, I didn't remain well for long. Just when I would think I was getting better, I would get worse again suddenly, as if I were being caught in storms or squalls that would come upon me unexpectedly.

The ups and downs of my condition started wearing me down psychologically, and I started becoming more careless. It was at that point that friends came to my rescue. It was only with their support that I was able to weather the storm. Through the combination of rest, the support of friends, and medication, I was finally able to felt constant, intense stress. I fell into depression's trap.

And a truly devious trap it is for, at first, I did not notice that I was trapped. I simply felt like something was different. I was more easily tired, I couldn't sleep, and I started having trouble concentrating. Still, I didn't even imagine that I could possibly have fallen into depression. I was busy, and I was thinking only of work, work, work. At some point, I started being less and less happy, and more and more anxious. I couldn't make decisions that had to be made. I would brood over things. Then I would think to myself "well, it'll just take care of itself, somehow," and I wouldn't do anything, so naturally the problem would get worse, and before too long it was affecting my work as well as my private life.

It finally occurred to me that I might be in trouble - that I might be developing depression - and I started to take an antidepressant. I thought that I would get better if I just made sure to take my medicine. Even this was a commendable level of resolve for me, since normally I am pretty bad even about taking prescription medicine that I only have to take for a few short days, and I am not very good about following doctors' orders. Just taking any medicine at all seemed to me like a last resort. I left my treatment entirely to the medicine, and continued working. At any rate, I was incredibly busy – I didn't have time to get sick. However, on top of making the terrible mistake of not taking time off to rest, a close friend of mine died suddenly, and the additional, intense shock of that event

Preface

This is the story of a psychiatrist suffering from depression. I hope that by reading this story the reader will gain a better understanding of the nature of this illness. However, this story does not unfold in strictly chronological order, so I have added this preface to provide a supplementary explanation to allow the reader to follow the story more easily.

This is my story - that is, I am the psychiatrist who became depressed. I have close to 20 years of clinical experience in the field of psychiatry, and have also been involved in educational and research activities. It is rumored that physicians are fated to develop the illnesses in which they specialize, but I thought that was only said about world-class researchers who were totally engrossed in their work, so I didn't think it would apply to me. Even so, sometimes I would daydream about what it would be like to come down with some sort of mental illness, but I never even wanted to daydream about coming down with depression, because I had seen firsthand the tremendous pain endured by people suffering from depression.

However, for whatever reason, through some trick of fate I was stricken with the disease of which I was the most afraid. I developed chronic, persistent fatigue, and

to say." In several instances, I revised the Japanese after reading the English translation.

I would also like to thank the president of Seiwa Publishers, Mr. Yuji Ishizawa, my editor, Ms. Yuko Sone and the designer, Ms. Yumiko Takayama; without their support, this book would have never been published. Mr. Ishizawa and Ms. Sone respected and took very seriously my desire to be of some help, however small, to the great number of people suffering from depression. I cannot thank them enough.

didn't use a tape recorder, but I did resolve to take notes, to the extent that I was able, in outline format. Doing this helped me greatly for, even when it seemed as if I would be swallowed up by my symptoms, writing them down helped me to consciously distance myself, and observe my symptoms as objectively as possible. This greatly eased my pain.

Mark Thorpe not only designed the cover page and provided the photographs that appear in this book, but also advised and supported me greatly on a personal level, as well. The title of this book, "*an ordinary psychiatrist? – navigating the darkness of depression –*," was also his idea. He was also recently awarded the "Prix du Public" (Public Prize) for his latest film, "The Majesty of Muck," at 34^e Festival Mondial de L'Image Sous-Marine (the 34th World Festival of Underwater Pictures), which was held in Antibes, France.

Lee Dancy took the time to figure out what I was trying to say, even when I couldn't come up with the proper expressions myself, in order to put my story into English. I want to thank him for the tremendous amount of time he spent working with me to refine my initial draft into the form in which it has now been published. There were many times when I myself was not really be happy with the Japanese I had written. Then I would read the English translation and think "Of course – that's what I was *trying*

Acknowledgements

In Japan, since 1998, there have been more than 30,000 completed suicides every year, which means that there are more deaths due to suicide than to automobile accidents. Although there are many contributing factors, including societal factors, the level of awareness of clinical depression among the population at large is still low, many people with clinical depression are going without treatment, and there is still lingering prejudice with respect to mental illness and psychiatric care. Wonderful books have been published in Japan by experts aiming to explain clinical depression to the layperson. While there thus may be no need for me to write one more such book, it is my hope that this book may be of some use to a wide range of people, including people who are suffering from clinical depression.

I am indebted to many people for helping me write this book, including Mark Thorpe, my coauthor, and Lee Dancy, for translating the original Japanese into English. I would like to express my sincerest thanks to Dr. Sakai, for recommending that I keep a written record of the symptoms I experienced. When I complained that I would not be able to sit down at my computer and maintain my concentration long enough to keep such a diary, he suggested dictating into a tape recorder. In the end, I

an ordinary psychiatrist?
– navigating the darkness of depression –

by **akemi**

photos and captions by **mark thorpe**

english translation by **lee dancy**

©2007 by Akemi and Mark Thorpe

an ordinary psychiatrist?
– navigating the darkness of depression –

First published on November 20, 2007

author	**akemi**
photos and captions	**mark thorpe**
english translation	**lee dancy**
publisher	**yuji ishizawa**
	Seiwa Shoten Publishers
	1-2-5 Kamitakaido,
	Suginami-ku
	Tokyo 168-0074, Japan
	Phone 03-3329-0031
	(Sales Department)
	03-3329-0033
	(Editorial Department)
	Fax 03-5374-7186
	http//www.seiwa-pb.co.jp

普通の精神科医？
－うつ病の闇への航海－

2007年11月20日　初版第1刷発行

著　　者	明　海
写真・解説	マーク・ソープ
翻　　訳	リー・ダンシー
発　行　者	石澤雄司
発　行　所	株式会社星和書店
	東京都杉並区上高井戸
	1－2－5　〒168-0074
	電話 03(3329)0031　（営業）
	03(3329)0033　（編集）
	FAX 03(5374)7186
	http://www.seiwa-pb.co.jp

Printed in Japan　ISBN978-4-7911-0648-6

an ordinary psychiatrist?
– navigating the darkness of depression –

by **akemi**

photos and captions by **mark thorpe**

english translation by **lee dancy**

©2007 by Akemi and Mark Thorpe